The Eggplant Cancer Cure

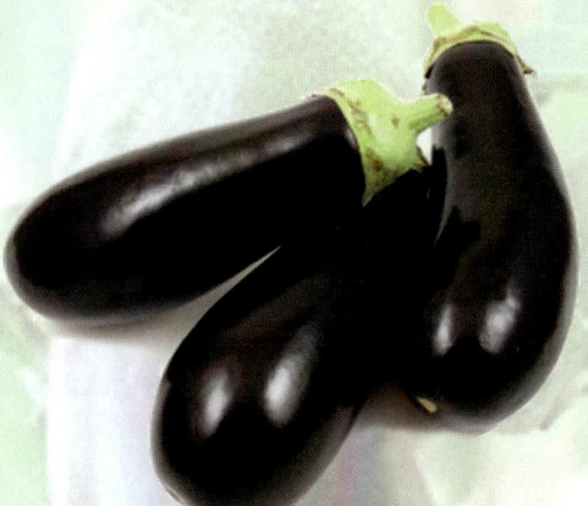

A Treatment for Skin Cancer
and
New Hope for Other Cancers
from Nature's Pharmacy

Dr. Bill E. Cham, Ph.D.

Smart Publications™
www.smart-publications.com

The Eggplant Cancer Cure

Dr. Bill E. Cham Ph.D.

Published by:

Smart Publications™

PO Box 4667
Petaluma, CA 94955
www.smart-publications.com

Published in the United States of America
First Edition, 2007

Library of Congress Control Number: 2007933714

ISBN: 1-890572-21-7 978-1-890572-21-1 Hardcover

Warning—Disclaimer

Smart Publications™ has designed this book to provide information in regard to the subject matter covered. It is sold with the understanding that the publisher and the author are not liable for the misconception or misuse of the information provided. Every effort has been to make this book as complete and as accurate as possible. The purpose of this book is to educate and entertain. The author and Smart Publications™ shall have neither liability nor responsibility to any person or entity with respect to any loss, damage caused, or alleged to have been caused, directly or indirectly, by the information contained in this book.

This book is dedicated to my family: Anita, Tania, Kai, Aruba, Karim, Georgie, Lane and Jessica.

Special thanks to Tania for her incredible dedication to finding relevant research papers and typing this manuscript and to Aruba for creating the artwork.

Also thanks to my co-investigators and all the patients who have encouraged the execution of the research and made it all worthwhile.

FOREWORD

Perfection or near-perfection is rare in any area of medicine. Dr. Bill Cham has achieved it in the treatment of two common cancers, basal cell carcinoma and squamous cell carcinoma. Dr. Cham's treatment also eliminates actinic keratosis, a usually benign (but potentially malignant) skin condition of middle ages and older.

What's near-perfection? A treatment that:

- Works nearly every time
- Is incredibly simple to use
- Has no adverse side effects
- Is inexpensive compared with other treatments

Even better, for those who want to know "how does it work", this book tells us exactly how. The explanation is simple, easy to understand, and yet scientifically elegant, a molecular ballet. Here's the explanation in one line of simple English: *Dr. Cham has found substances which can penetrate and kill skin cancer cells but can't penetrate normal skin cells, so normal skin cells are untouched and unhurt while the skin cancer cells die!* (Those who want the full technical explanation will find it — again, in simple English — in the following pages.)

What you're about to read and the pictures you're about to see are absolutely breath-taking. You'll read about and see relatively small squamous and basal cell cancers disappearing in just 12 to 16 weeks. You'll see large, neglected cancers as large as 2 by 3 inches first get bigger as cancer cells "beneath the surface" die, and then reverse course and slowly heal over the next few months. Surgical treatment of such large skin cancers is almost always disfiguring, and sometimes not correctable with plastic surgery. Dr. Cham's treatment enables healing of even the largest cancers with minimal if any disfigurement.

So where's this treatment been? Why haven't you heard about it from your doctor? It's been used for years in Australia, where it simultaneously cured approximately 70,000 Australians of their skin cancers and incurred the wrath of the Australasian College of Dermatologists and the (Australian) Therapeutic Goods Administration, neither of whom favor freedom of choice in health care, and have a special disinterest in un-"approved" therapies. But enough about that —"fans" of the Food and Drug Administration in these United States are more than familiar with this situation.

Always work with a physician skilled and knowledgeable in natural medicine. Ask him or her where to find Dr. Cham's skin cancer cure. In a "wired world", you can also enter "curadermglobal.com", "Curaderm" or "BEC-5" into your search engine, and proceed accordingly. Remember, Dr. Cham's treatment can cure squamous cell cancer, basal cell cancer, and actinic keratosis but not melanoma. Also, it may not work on skin cancers that have already undergone surgery. But given these precautions, **Dr. Cham has discovered, and then thoroughly researched and developed a near-perfect treatment for two common skin cancers. If anyone deserves a Nobel Prize in Medicine, it's Dr. Bill E. Cham.**

jonathan v. wright, m.d.

medical director, tahoma clinic
renton, washington, usa
www.tahomaclinic.com
www.wrightnewsletter.com

Books authored or co-authored by Dr. Wright include Book of Nutritional Therapy (1979), Guide to Healing with Nutrition (1984), The Natural Pharmacy (1994), Natural Hormone Replacement for Women over 45 (1997), Maximize Your Vitality and Potency for Men Over 40 (1999), Why Stomach Acid is Good for You (2001), D-Mannose & Bladder Infection (2002), Prevent Tooth Decay with Xylitol (2003), Thriving Through Dialysis (2005), Natural Medicine, Optimal Wellness (2006)

TABLE OF CONTENTS

CHAPTER 3:

CHAPTER 4:

CHAPTER 5:

PROLOGUE

THE "MUTILATED MAN"

Sometime ago, in the 1990s, there was a knock on my door. "Come in," I said. The door opened slowly, an elderly couple entered. The male had a veil covering his face and hat on his head. The lady said, "Sorry doctor but can we see you for a moment"? I agreed and both sat down. The lady said, "We saw you and some patients you treated for skin cancer on TV several weeks ago. In particular we were impressed by the segment which showed how your treatment saved the nose of the patient who had skin cancer. We are here to encourage you and support your work. I would like to show you why we are so interested in helping you and others. This is my husband." She then asked him to remove his veil and hat. I could not believe my eyes. His head was disfigured. He had no nose, both ears were gone, one eye was half closed, there were large indented areas with transplanted skin on his head and half his chin was gone. I felt so sorry for the man. Choked, I attempted to say, "How did this happen?" "It is all skin cancer," the man said. "Over the years I have had skin cancers that were treated by radiotherapy and surgery and this is the end result. I have been mutilated." He was quick to point out that he did not blame the radiotherapist or surgeon for his afflictions, but he felt it was time that a better treatment was made available for the general public. "The lady you treated as shown on the TV would have probably ended up like me in several years time. Although it is too late for me, I want to help other people by not having to go through what I am going through. One of my latest treated skin cancers has now traveled through my body and cannot be treated. So, we are here to stimulate you to continue your work and to congratulate you on your achievements." I felt so humble and grateful. This showed unselfishness, and compassion beyond expression. The conversation ended soon after. Several weeks later I had a telephone call from the lady who informed me that her husband had passed away. I have never forgotten this experience and this, amongst other events, has inspired me to ensure that my attention was directed to continue my tireless quest for a better treatment for skin cancers.

the treatment of skin cancers.

Twenty five years of basic research, pre-clinical research and clinical research have established that BEC, at lower concentrations than is present in the eggplant, in a cream formulation now available to the public known as Curaderm BEC5, is effective for treating non melanoma skin cancers. The glycoalkaloids in BEC are currently undergoing clinical trials in humans suffering from terminal internal cancers.

The objective of this book is to describe the scientific development of an anticancer drug that is extracted from an edible fruit, the eggplant.

In this book the words cancer cure has the medical definition of "a cancer is considered to be cured if it disappears and does not recur within five years." As you will read, patients were made healthy again by the eggplant treatment and were followed-up for over a decade after they were healed of their cancer and there were no recurrences.

When reading this book you will appreciate that no experimental short cuts were taken and the development of Curaderm BEC5 followed the necessary stringent pathways and time requirements which are essential before any new drug, natural or synthetic, can be safely marketed for certain indications.

This communication briefly describes in summarized form only, the essence of the 25 years of investigations. For more elaborate published scientific information please see the bibliography section in this book.

The photographic figures of treated lesions have not been modified or tampered with. They are all original.

Before the research and new treatments are described, a guide to cancer in general and skin cancer in particular are presented.

CANCER

Cancer develops when cells in a part of the body begin to grow out of control. Although there are many kinds of cancer, they all start because of out-of-control growth of abnormal cells which develop into malignant growths or tumours.

Normal body cells grow, divide, and die in an orderly fashion. During the early years of life, normal cells divide more rapidly until adulthood. After that, cells in most parts of the body divide only to replace worn-out or dying cells and to repair injuries.

Because cancer cells continue to grow and divide, they are different from normal cells. Instead of dying, they outlive normal cells and continue to form new abnormal cells.

Cancer cells often travel to other parts of the body where they begin to grow and replace normal tissue. This process, called metastasis, occurs as the cancer cells get into the bloodstream or lymph vessels of our body.

Cancer cells develop because of damage to DNA. This substance is in every cell and directs all its activities. Most of the time when DNA becomes damaged the body is able to repair it. In cancer cells, the damaged DNA is not repaired. People can inherit damaged DNA, which accounts for inherited cancers. Many times though, a person's DNA becomes damaged by exposure to something in the environment, like smoking or over-exposure of UV radiation.

Cancer usually forms as a tumour. Some cancers, like leukemia, do not form tumours. Instead, these cancer cells involve the blood and blood-forming organs, and circulate through other tissues where they grow.
Not all tumours are cancerous. Benign (noncancerous) tumours do not spread to other parts of the body (metastasize) and, with very rare exceptions, are not life-threatening.

Different types of cancer can behave very differently. For example, lung cancer and skin cancer are very different diseases. They grow at different rates and respond to different treatments. That is why people with cancer need treatment that is aimed at their particular kind of cancer.

Cancer is the second leading cause of death in the United States. Half of all men and one-third of all women in the US will develop cancer during their lifetimes. Today, millions of people are living with cancer or have had cancer. The risk of developing most types of cancer can be reduced by changes in a person's lifestyle, for example, by quitting smoking, protecting against UV damage and eating a better diet. The sooner a cancer is found and treatment begins, the better are the chances for living for many years.

Lesions of the Skin

Actinic Keratoses and other Precancers

A number of abnormal but relatively harmless skin growths constitute the early warning signs of skin cancer. These may be precancerous lesions, benign tumours that mask or mimic more serious ones, or malignant tumours that are at the moment just on the topmost layer of the skin. They are important to recognize, because they are a warning sign of potential skin cancer.

Precancerous Growths

Skin in a precancerous state is abnormal but not malignant. The term "precancerous" is used because these abnormal areas of skin are more likely to turn malignant than healthy skin. Precancerous growths are visible to the naked eye, and they look different from normal cells when they are examined under a microscope.

Early Cancer

When malignant changes occur to the skin, but haven't spread beyond the top layer of the skin, they are called early cancers, or cancers *in situ*. A barrier called the basement membrane helps delay invasion by malignant cells deeper into the skin.

Types of Precancer

Actinic Keratosis

Actinic keratosis (AK), also known as solar keratosis, is the result of prolonged exposure to sunlight. It is a small crusty, scaly or crumbly bump or horn that arises on the skin surface. The base may be light or dark, tan, pink, red, or a combination of these lesions or the same colour as your skin. The scale or crust is horny, dry, and rough, and is often recognized by touch rather than sight. Occasionally it itches or produces a pricking or tender sensation. It can also become inflamed and surrounded by redness. In rare instances, actinic keratoses can bleed.

The skin abnormality or lesion develops slowly and usually reaches a size from an eighth to a quarter of an inch (2mm to 4mm) but can sometimes be as large as one inch. Early on, it may disappear only to reappear later. It is not unusual to see several AKs at a time. AKs most likely appear on the face, lips, ears, scalp, neck, backs of the hands and forearms, shoulders and back — the parts of the body most often exposed to sunshine. The growths may be flat and pink or raised and rough.

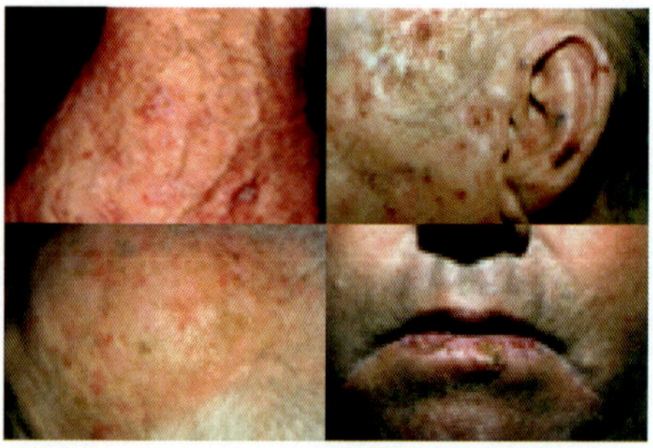

Fig. 1-1: Actinic Keratoses

Actinic Cheilitis

Actinic cheilitis is a type of actinic keratosis occurring on the lips. It causes them to become dry, cracked, scaly and pale or white. It mainly affects the lower lip, which typically receives more sun exposure than the upper lip.

Arsenical Keratosis

Far less common, arsenical keratosis is an accumulation of keratinized tissue that at first resembles numerous small, yellowish corns. These arise most often on the palms, soles, and inner surfaces of the finger and toes, and then enlarge and thicken, sometimes increasing in number. Although rarely seen today, arsenical keratoses usually occur on patients who were at some time in their lives exposed to arsenic, either contained in medication or from an industrial or environmental source.

Leukoplakia

Leukoplakia is a disease of the mucous membrane. White patches or plaques develop on the tongue or inside of the mouth, and have the ability to develop into SCC. It is caused by sources of continuous irritation, including smoking or other tobacco use, rough teeth or rough edges on dentures and fillings. Leukoplakia on the lips is mainly caused by sun damage.

Bowen's Disease

This is generally considered to be a superficial SCC that has not yet spread. It appears as a persistent red–brown, scaly patch which may resemble psoriasis or eczema. If untreated, it may invade deeper structures.

Skin Cancer

Skin cancer is a disease in which skin cells lose the ability to divide and grow normally. Healthy skin cells normally divide in an orderly way to replace dead cells and grow new skin. Abnormal cells can grow out of control and form a mass or 'tumour'. When abnormal cells originate in the skin, the mass is called a skin tumour.

A skin tumour is considered benign if it is limited to a few cell layers and does not invade surrounding tissues or organs. But if the tumour spreads to surrounding tissues it is considered malignant or cancerous.

Cancer cells crowd out and destroy nearby healthy cells forming growths called malignant tumours.

Most skin growths, however, are non-malignant, benign (not harmful) tumours.

- Some forms of skin cancer also metastasize. That is, they spread to other parts of the body and start new tumours.
- Skin cancer that spreads to vital organs like the brain or liver can be life threatening.

The skin, which is the human body's largest organ, has several functions. It prevents the body from losing water and other fluids, stores fat, cools the body when sweat evaporates, and makes vitamin D. The skin also protects the body from infection, light, and injury.

There are three layers of skin:

1. Epidermis - the outer layer of skin
2. Dermis - the middle layer of the skin; contains nerves, blood vessels, sweat glands, hair follicles, and oil-producing cells that keep the skin from drying out
3. Fatty layer - the deep layer of skin

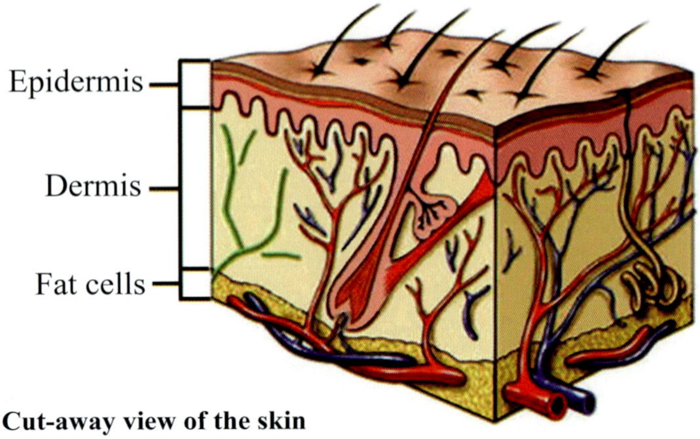

Fig. 1-2: Cut-away view of the skin

Skin cancer begins in the epidermis, the outer layer of skin. The epidermis has three kinds of cells.

- Squamous cells are cells that progressively flatten and fill with protective keratin (a tough, insoluble protein that makes skin almost completely waterproof) to form the outmost surface of the skin.
- Basal cells are small cells located at the base of the epidermis that serve as a reservoir for squamous cells shed from the skin.
- Melanocytes are cells that produce a dark material, or pigment, that gives the skin its colour.

Each of these cells can suddenly start to divide abnormally and become cancerous. The main types of skin cancer are named after these cells.

SYMPTOMS OF SKIN CANCER

Skin cancer first appears as a growth, or abnormal accumulation of cells. It sometimes takes the form of a sore or pimple that does not heal. The sore may bleed or ooze fluid, crust or scab over, and then ooze or bleed again. Cancer can occur on almost any area of the skin, but is most common on areas often exposed to the sun. Skin cancer usually is painless.

The most common symptoms are:

- A new growth on the skin.
- A change in an existing skin growth.
- A sore that does not heal.

Not all changes in the skin are symptoms of skin cancer.

DIFFERENT TYPES OF SKIN CANCER

There are a number of different types of skin cancers depending on the type of skin cell from which they arise. Each kind of skin cancer has its own distinctive appearance. Certain skin cancers also tend to develop in specific areas of the body.

- Basal cell carcinoma.
- Squamous cell carcinoma.
- A third type, malignant melanoma, is relatively rare but can be very dangerous.

BASAL CELL CARCINOMA

Basal cell carcinoma (BCC) is the most common form of cancer, with more than one million new cases estimated in the US each year. Basal cells are cells that line the deepest layer of the epidermis. An abnormal growth — a tumour — of this layer is known as basal cell carcinoma.

Basal cell carcinoma can usually be diagnosed with a simple biopsy and is fairly easy to treat when detected early. However, 5 to 10 percent of BCCs can be resistant to treatment or locally aggressive, eating away at the skin around them, sometimes even into bone and cartilage. When not treated quickly, they can be difficult to eliminate. Fortunately, however, this is a cancer that has an extremely low rate of metastasis, and although it can result in scars and disfigurement, it is not usually life-threatening.

There are five most typical characteristics of basal cell carcinoma which are shown below. Frequently, two or more features are present in one tumour. In addition, BCC sometimes resembles non-cancerous skin conditions such as psoriasis or eczema.

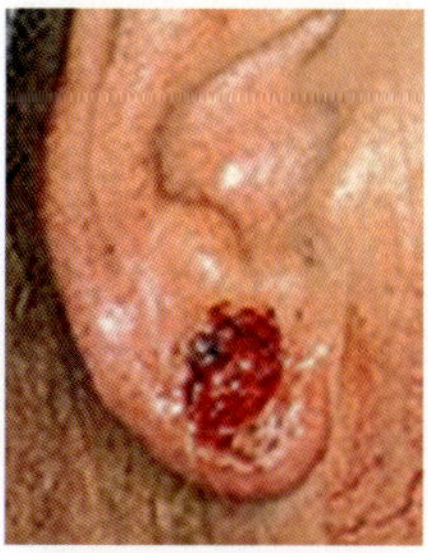

An Open Sore that bleeds, oozes, or crusts and remains open for three or more weeks. A persistent, non-healing sore is a very common sign of an early basal cell carcinoma.

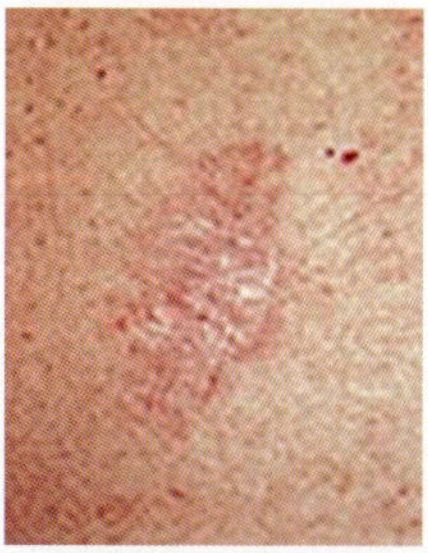

A Reddish Patch or irritated area, frequently occurring on the chest, shoulders, arms, or legs. Sometimes the patch crusts. It may also itch or hurt. At other times, it persists with no noticeable discomfort.

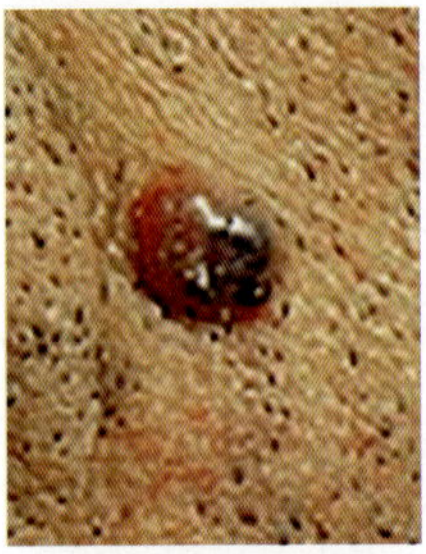

A Shiny Bump or nodule that is pearly or translucent and is often pink, red, or white. The bump can also be tan, black, or brown, especially in dark-haired people, and can be confused with a mole.

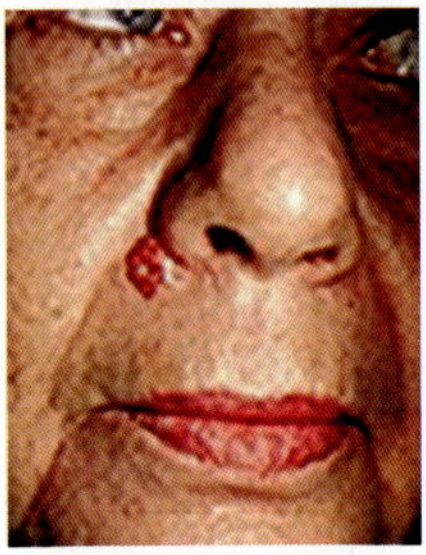

A Pink Growth with a slightly elevated rolled border and a crusted indentation in the center. As the growth slowly enlarges, tiny blood vessels may develop on the surface.

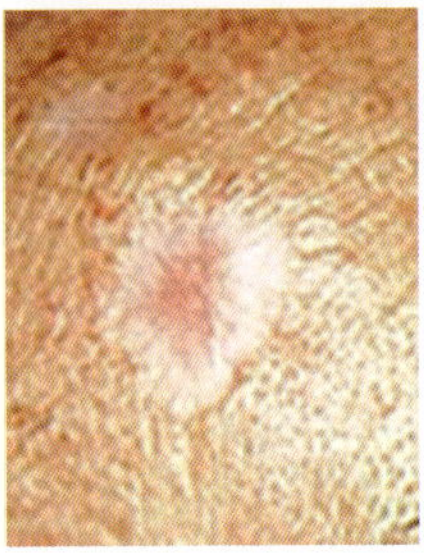

A Scar-like Area which is white, yellow or waxy, and often has poorly defined borders. The skin itself appears shiny and taut. This warning sign can indicate the presence of an aggressive tumour.

Fig. 1-3: Various BCCs

TYPES OF BASAL CELL CARCINOMA

Nodular. Nodular basal cell carcinoma is the most common type. This tumour usually resembles a smooth, round, waxy pimple, pale yellow or pearl gray, and may vary in size from a few millimeters to 1 centimeter. Often, the skin covering the nodule is so thin that the slightest injury will cause it to bleed. These tumours are often depressed in the middle and show ulceration. As the tumour grows, it destroys healthy structures in its path, including nerves, muscles, and blood vessels. Large tumours are easily diagnosed, but smaller ones are often difficult to tell from benign skin conditions, such as warts, seborrheic keratoses, moles, psoriasis, or fever sores.

Superficial. This is a less common type of BCC. It is a progressively spreading, slow growing cancer that differs greatly from other types of this disease. The tumour is red, with a slightly raised ulcerated or crusted surface, often bordered with pearly or threadlike formations. Tumours usually appear as patches on the torso, but can develop more extensively on the face and neck. This is often mistaken for other skin conditions such as fungal infections, eczema, or psoriasis.

Morpheoic, Sclerosing or Fibrosing. Fibrosing basal cell carcinoma is also called morphea-like carcinoma. This fibrosing type of tumour begins as a flat or slightly depressed, shiny, hard, yellow-white patch with an irregular border. Sometimes, it may be present for years without growing or changing or being recognized. Usually, though, the lesion grows quickly, reaching a diameter of several centimeters within a few months. This is a fairly uncommon type of skin cancer, and can be difficult to eradicate because of root-like extensions of the tumour that reach into the underlying tissue.

Pigmented. Pigmented basal cell carcinoma is similar to nodular basal cell carcinoma, but is more likely to appear in people with dark hair or dark eyes. As its name implies, this growth is almost black and can easily be mistaken for the more aggressive malignant melanoma.

SQUAMOUS CELL CARCINOMA

Squamous cell carcinoma is the second most common form of skin cancer, with over 200,000 new cases per year estimated in the United States, and about 1,900 deaths from this type of cancer. Squamous cells are cells that compose most of the epidermis. An abnormal growth of these cells is known as a squamous cell carcinoma.

TYPES OF SQUAMOUS CELL CARCINOMA

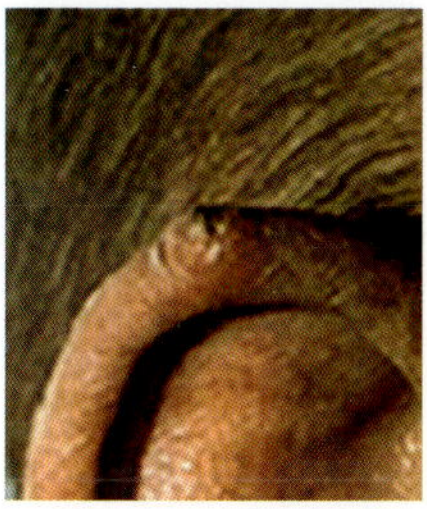

A wart-like growth that crusts and occasionally bleeds.

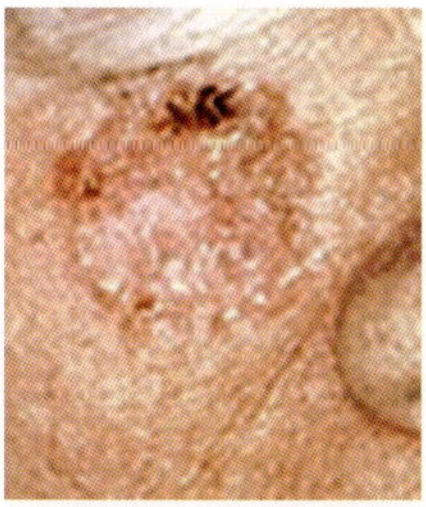

A persistent, scaly red patch with irregular borders that sometimes crusts or bleeds.

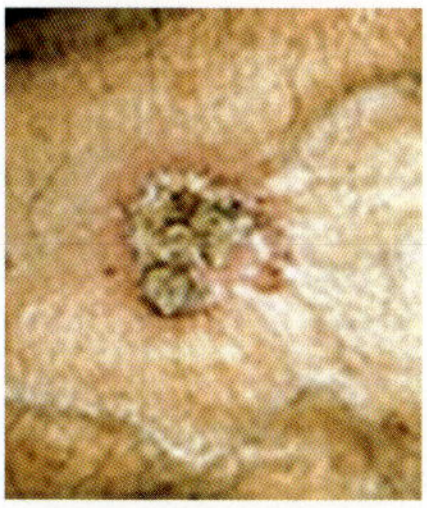

An open sore that bleeds and crusts and persists for weeks.

TYPES OF SQUAMOUS CELL CARCINOMA CONTINUTED

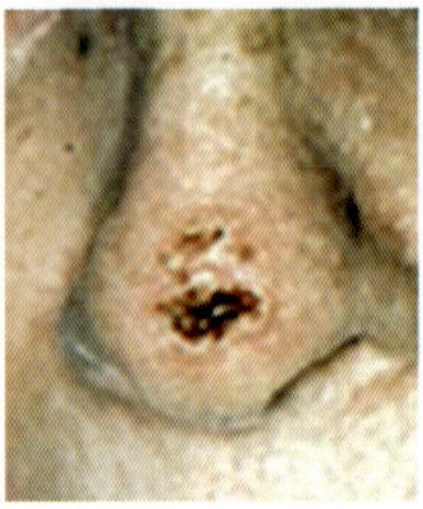

An elevated growth with a central depression that occasionally bleeds. A growth of this type may rapidly increase in size.

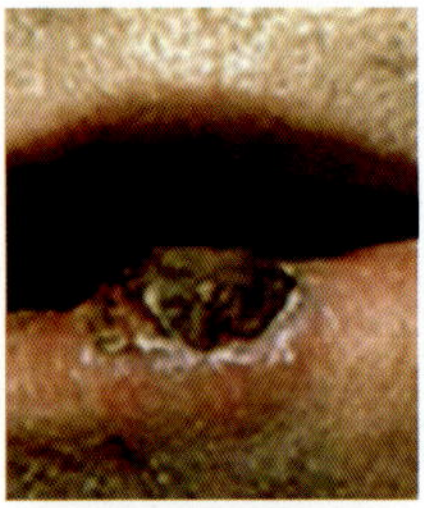

A persistent, scaly red patch with irregular borders that sometimes crusts or bleeds.

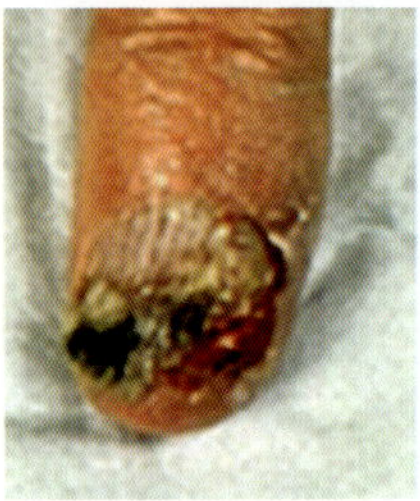

An open sore that bleeds and crusts and persists for weeks.

Fig. 1-4: Various SCCs

Likely Places Where Skin Cancers Develop

Basal cell carcinomas usually occur on parts of the body that are often exposed to the sun. These are the face, neck, V-shaped area of the chest, and upper back. They occur less often on the top sides of the arms and hands.

- These tumours sometimes look like a sore or pimple that does not heal.
- They may ooze yellowish fluid, crust over with a scab, and then break down and ooze again.
- When the surrounding skin is stretched, a basal cell carcinoma has a pearly gray look, with tiny blood vessels often visible inside the tumour.

Squamous cell carcinomas also appear most often on the face and neck, V-shaped area of the chest, and upper back. They are more likely than basal cell carcinomas to form on the top of the arms and hands.

- Squamous cell carcinomas look like an inflamed (pink ish or reddish), scaly growth that feels sore or tender.
- Some may repeatedly break open, bleed, and crust - never fully healing.

Chapter 2

WHAT CAUSES SKIN CANCER

There is convincing evidence that sunlight causes skin cancer.

The types of sun radiation include:

- visible light, which gives us the colours we see,
- infrared radiation which gives us the warmth we feel, and
- ultraviolet (UV) radiation.

Ultraviolet (UV) radiation can cause harmful effects to the skin.

There are three basic types of ultraviolet radiation:

- UVA (long-wave UV),
- UVB (sunburn UV), and
- UVC (short-wave UV).

Table 2-1 summarizes the general features of each type.

Table 2-1
Types of Ultraviolet Radiation and Their Features

Ultraviolet Radiation Type	General Features
Ultraviolet A radiation (UVA, long-wave UV)	-not filtered out in the atmosphere -passes through glass -produces some tanning -once considered harmless but now believed harmful over the long term -levels remain relatively constant throughout the day -causes premature ageing of the skin, wrinkling

Ultraviolet Radiation Type	General Features
Ultraviolet B radiation (UVB, sunburn radiation)	-some filtered out in the atmosphere by the ozone layer -does not pass through glass -causes sunburn, tanning, wrinkling, ageing of the skin and skin cancer -highest intensity at noontime
Ultraviolet C radiation (UVC, short-wave UV)	-filtered out in the atmosphere by the ozone layer before reaching earth -major artificial sources are germicidal lamps -burns the skin and causes skin cancer

Table 2-1

The effects of sunlight on the skin

When ultraviolet radiation reaches the skin, some radiation is reflected away from the surface. The remaining radiation is scattered into the tissues just beneath the skin's surface. A fraction of this radiation is absorbed by the skin's living cells.

Ultraviolet radiation absorbed by living cells damages sensitive substances that influence the skin's normal growth and appearance. Damage can result in:

- sunburn,
- increased rate of ageing of the skin, and
- skin cancer.

Sunburn

Sunburn is the most familiar and immediate effect of ultraviolet radiation on the skin. It is an inflammation caused by an increase in bloodflow beneath the skin. The reaction is not normally instantaneous, but reaches a bright red colour within 15 to 20 hours. The condition can be very painful and sometimes causes peeling of the skin.

Brief intense exposure can cause severe sunburn in people who are not accustomed to strong sunlight. There is evidence that this type of exposure, as well as long-term exposures, might be linked to serious forms of skin cancer later in life. Usually five sunburns over a period of time will cause skin cancer.

Increased Rate of Ageing of the Skin

Repeated exposure to the sun's ultraviolet radiation eventually causes skin damage similar to the ageing process. Patches of skin become thin and less elastic, and develop blemishes, sun freckles, and wrinkles. These changes may take many years of exposure but when they occur, the damage is irreversible.

Skin Cancer

If exposure to sunlight continues for several years, the damaged skin has an increased chance of developing one of the forms of skin cancer. Exposure to ultraviolet radiation increases the risk of developing these cancers (although it may not be the only cause of the disease). While the exact relationship is not entirely defined, it appears that intermittent (occasional) exposure and exposure during childhood and adolescence are likely important predictors for basal cell carcinoma and cutaneous malignant melanoma. High levels of chronic exposure, such as working outdoors, is more often associated with squamous cell tumours.

The following facts also link sunlight exposure to skin cancer:

- Most skin cancer occurs in areas of skin most heavily exposed to sunlight (ears, forehead, arms, etc).
- Skin cancer among people who are sensitive to sunlight is more common in regions with stronger sunlight.
- People with genetic diseases that make them more sensitive to sunlight have a greater chance of developing skin cancer.
- Studies show that ultraviolet radiation similar to sunlight causes skin cancer in animals.

- UV radiation from tanning beds, or from sun lamps may cause skin cancer. While skin cancer has been associated with sunburn, moderate tanning may also produce the same effect. UV radiation can also have a damaging effect on the immune system and cause premature ageing of the skin, giving it a wrinkled, leathery appearance.

Types of skin cancer linked to sunlight exposure

Three different types of skin cancer are linked to sunlight exposure:

- basal cell cancer,
- squamous cell cancer, and
- malignant melanoma.

Factors affecting risks of developing skin cancer

Five main factors influence the risk of skin cancer:

- skin pigment and ability to tan,
- heredity,
- exposure to chemicals,
- amount of exposure to sunlight, and
- people who have had organ transplants and are on immuno-suppressive drugs are prone to developing squamous cell carcinoma.

Skin Pigment and Ability to Tan

Ultraviolet radiation from sunlight affects everybody's skin to some extent, but the skin's response varies widely from person to person. People's sensitivity to the sun varies according to the amount of pigment in the skin and the skin's ability to tan.

Ultraviolet radiation causes tanning in two different ways: by immediate tanning and by delayed tanning. Immediate tanning causes the skin to darken in response to UVA. This darkening begins during the period of exposure, but fades within a few hours or days. The amount of tanning increases according to the skin's natural darkness and previous amount of tanning.

Delayed tanning occurs two to three days after exposure to either UVA or UVB. It lasts from several weeks to months, and is maintained by repeated exposure to sunlight. With delayed tanning, the skin increases its production and distribution of dark pigment. The skin also becomes thicker. These changes can follow sunburning or develop gradually over a long period of repeated brief exposures to sunlight.

Some people burn easily after the first hour of sun exposure following winter or any period away from the sun. Other people, especially those with dark skin, never burn. This difference in reaction makes it possible to classify skin into one of six different types (see Table 2-2).

Table 2-2
Classification of Skin Types

Skin Type	Hair	Complexion	Freckles	Sun Reaction	Tanning
I	Red or Blond	very fair	+++	always burns	never tans
II	Blond	fair	++	often burns	tans lightly
III	Blond or Light Brown	fair to medium	+ to 0	sometimes burns	tans progressively
IV	Brown	Olive	0	rarely burns	tans easily
V	Brown to Black	dark	0	rarely burns	tans deeply
VI	Black	very dark	0	never burns	tans deeply

The risk of skin cancer from the sun generally follows the same pattern. Darker skinned people have lower risk of sun-induced skin cancer. The person most prone to skin cancer caused by sunlight tans poorly and suffers sunburn easily. Frequent and/or intense sunburn in children with fair skin and freckles has been linked to malignant melanoma later in life.

Heredity

For reasons not completely understood, people with Celtic heritage (Irish, Scottish or Northern European) have increased risk of skin cancer from the sun. Genetic diseases that affect the skin can also increase the risk. For example, albinism, a genetic condition which prevents the production of normal skin pigments, makes the skin sensitive to ultraviolet light.

Exposure to Chemicals

Exposure to certain chemicals can increase the skin's sensitivity to ultraviolet light through a process called photosensitization. Examples of such chemicals include:

- coal tar pitch and petroleum products containing polycyclic aromatic hydrocarbons (PAHs),
- certain printing chemicals used in photosensitive printing processes,
- certain drugs and antibiotics such as tetracyclines, sulfonamides, thiazide diuretics, chlorpromazine, oral contraceptives, and
- chemicals called psoralens found naturally in certain plants, fruits and vegetables.

Antibiotics must be taken internally before the skin becomes sensitive to sunlight. However, simple skin contact with psoralens, which are found in figs, parsnips, citrus plants, or moldy celery, can make the skin more susceptible to sunburns in some individuals.

Immuno-Compromised Organ Transplant Patients

Organ transplant patients usually take immuno-suppressive drugs to reduce the body's rejection of the transplanted organ. Suppression of the immune system by heavy doses of drugs after transplant surgery contribute to the incidence of skin cancer. Approximately 35 to 70 percent of organ transplant patients develop skin cancer within 20 years following transplant surgery, depending on geographic location. Some transplant recipients have more than 100 squamous cell carcinomas a year. More alarmingly, some long-term transplant patients actually die from skin cancer.

Chapter 3

PREVIOUS ACCEPTED TREATMENTS

ACTINIC KERATOSIS

There is no one best method to treat all skin cancers and precancers. The choice is determined by many factors, including the location, type, size, whether it is a primary tumour or a recurrent one, and also health and preference of the patient. For example, a treatment that has a high cure rate and is painless but leaves a large scar might not be preferred for a tumour on the face.

Almost all treatments are performed in the physician's office or in special surgical facilities. Most skin cancer removal can be done using a local anaesthetic. Rarely, extensive tumours may require general anaesthesia and hospital admission.

There are many methods for eliminating AKs. All cause a certain amount of reddening, and some may cause scarring, while other approaches are less likely to do so.

Cryosurgery

The most common treatment for AKs, it is especially effective when a limited number of lesions exist. Liquid nitrogen is applied to the growths with a spray device or cotton-tipped applicator to freeze them. They subsequently shrink or become crusted and fall off, without requiring any cutting or anaesthesia. Some temporary redness and swelling may occur after treatment, and in dark-skinned patients, some pigment may be lost.

Curettage and Desiccation

This procedure is for lesions suspected to be early cancers. To test for malignancy, the physician takes a biopsy specimen, either by shaving off the top of the lesion with a scalpel or scraping it off with a curette. Then the curette is used to remove the base of the lesion. Bleeding is stopped with an electrocautery needle, and local anaesthesia is required.

Topical Medications

Medicated creams and solutions are used to remove both visible and invisible AKs when the lesions are numerous. The patient applies the medication according to a schedule. After treatment, some discomfort may result from skin breakdown.

5-fluorouracil (5-FU) cream or solution, in concentrations from 0.5 to 5 percent, is the most widely used topical treatment for AK. It is used on the face, ears, and neck. Some redness, swelling, and crusting may occur.

Another preparation, imiquimod cream, is used for multiple keratoses. It causes cells to produce interferon, a chemical that destroys cancerous and precancerous cells.

An alternative treatment, a gel combining hyaluronic acid and the anti-inflammatory drug diclofenac, is also used.

Chemical Peeling

This method makes use of trichloroacetic acid (TCA) or a similar agent applied directly to the skin. The top skin layers slough off, usually replaced within seven days by new epidermis (the skin's outermost layer). This technique requires local anaesthesia and can cause temporary discolouration and irritation.

Laser Surgery

A carbon dioxide or erbium YAG laser is focused onto the lesion, removing epidermis and different amounts of deeper skin. This finely controlled treatment is an option for lesions in small or narrow areas; it can be effective for keratoses on the face and scalp, as well as actinic cheilitis on the lips. Laser surgery is useful for people with bleeding disorders and is also used as a secondary therapy when other techniques are unsuccessful. However, local anaesthesia is usually necessary, and some scarring and pigment loss can occur.

Photodynamic Therapy (PDT)

PDT may be used to treat lesions on the face and scalp. Topical *5-aminolevulinic acid* (5-ALA) is applied to the lesions by the physician. Within the next 24 hours, the medicated areas are exposed to strong light, which activates the 5-ALA. The treatment selectively destroys actinic keratoses, causing little damage to surrounding normal skin, although some swelling and redness often occur.

NON MELANOMA SKIN CANCERS

Treatment depends on the:

- type of skin cancer,
- its stage and location and the,
- individual's age and overall health.

People with small basal cell carcinomas, for instance, may need only simple treatment. That's because basal cell cancers rarely spread to other parts of the body and seldom are fatal. Squamous cell carcinomas have a greater tendency to spread, and may require more treatment.

Skin cancers are usually treated by a dermatologist, a doctor who specializes in skin diseases. Treatment often can be done in the doctor's office. Most require a local anaesthetic.

Some tiny skin cancers are completely removed during the biopsy. No more treatment is needed. However, most require additional treatment to eliminate all of the cancer cells.

Three kinds of treatment are used for most skin cancers. They are:

- Surgery: Taking out or destroying the cancer.
- Chemotherapy: Giving drugs to kill the cancer cells.
- Radiation therapy: Using powerful energy from x-rays or other sources to destroy the cancer cells.

In addition to these, there are other treatment options.

Surgery

Surgery is the most common treatment. Any of several surgical methods may be used:

- Simple excision involves cutting out the tumour with a margin of surrounding normal skin to be sure it is completely removed.
- Cryosurgery (cryo = "cold") freezes and kills the cancer cells. It uses liquid nitrogen, which has a temperature of 196 degrees below zero Celcius. The extreme cold instantly kills the tumour, which falls off like a scab after the area thaws. Cryosurgery itself is painless. However, the treated area may become swollen and painful after it thaws. Cryosurgery is used mainly for small or superficial skin cancers, and to remove precancerous growths.
- Curettage and electrodessication combines two methods. In one, the doctor uses a curette, a sharp, spoon-shaped instrument, to scoop out the tumour. The area is then treated with electrodessication, applying electrical current produced by a special machine. It controls bleeding, and dehydrates and kills cancer cells remaining near the edge of tumour area.
- Micrographic surgery (or Mohs surgery) attempts to remove all of the tumour and as little surrounding normal tissue as possible. One layer of tumour is removed and examined with a microscope. If cancer cells are present another layer is removed and examined. The process continues until all cancer cells have been removed.
- Laser surgery uses the highly focused beam of light from a laser to destroy cancer cells. It is seldom used for cancers that have not grown beyond the outer layer of the skin.
- Skin cancer surgery will leave a visible scar. Its size usually depends on the size of the cancer and the

amount of tissue removed during surgery.

- Cryosurgery for a small tumour usually leaves a faint, white scar.
- Treatment of large cancers may require a skin graft to close the defect. Grafting involves removing skin from another part of the body and moving it to the area where the cancer was removed.

Chemotherapy

Chemotherapy means treatment with anti-cancer drugs. The treatment for skin cancer often uses anti-cancer drugs in a lotion or cream applied to the skin. This localized, or topical, chemotherapy is for superficial tumours that have not advanced beyond the top layer of the skin.

Systemic chemotherapy also may be given in a pill, injected into a muscle, or intravenously through a needle in a vein. This body-wide, or systemic, chemotherapy can kill cancer cells that have spread outside the skin. It may cause nausea and other side effects in some individuals. Side effects are common. This treatment is generally used for metastatic cancer.

Radiation Therapy

Radiation therapy, or radiotherapy, uses a special kind of energy carried by invisible rays or particles to kill cancer cells, or keep them from growing. X-rays are the kind of radiation often used to kill skin cancer. The amounts are much higher than those used in an ordinary mammogram or chest x-ray. This therapy often is used for cancers that occur in areas difficult to treat with surgery, especially in the very elderly, who may be unable to safely undergo surgery. These include cancers on the ears, eyelids, and tip of the nose.

Radiation therapy may cause:

- Rash, redness, or dryness in the area.
- Other changes in skin texture or colour may develop after radiation therapy. They may become more noticeable years later.

RESEARCH

Research is the first step in biopharmaceutical product development. Initially this involves optimization of chemical structures into leading compounds. Once a leading compound has been identified, the pre-clinical phase commences.

BEC - Solasodine Glycosides

Our research has resulted in the identification and characterization of a mixture of solasodine glycosides consisting mainly of solasonine and solamargine from various plant sources including edible fruit such as the eggplant. The actives were termed BEC which is a standardized mixture of the two triglycosides, solasonine, solamargine and their corresponding di-and monoglycosides [5-15].

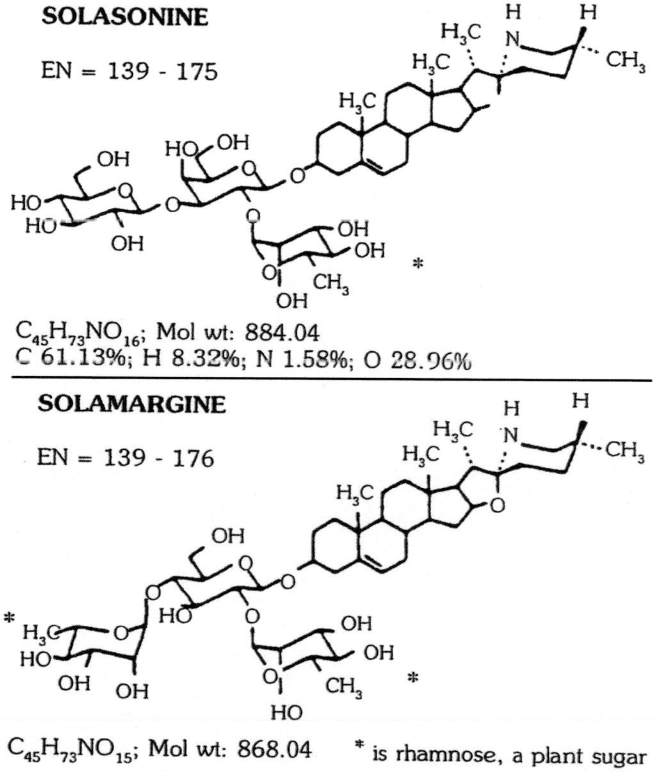

Fig. 4-2: BEC is a standardized mixture of sugar-bound Solasodine. The two main glycoalkaloids are Solasonine and Solamargine. All of the glycoalkaloids are made up of the steroid (aglycone meaning without sugar) Solasodine and one or more of the sugars rhamnose, glucose or galactose.

PRE-CLINICAL PHASE

In the pre-clinical phase, we evaluated BEC for possible therapeutic potential by conducting Ex vivo and In vivo studies.

Ex Vivo studies have demonstrated that BEC was effective against a wide spectrum of human cancers and that BEC was selectively killing cancer cells without harming normal cells [16-27].

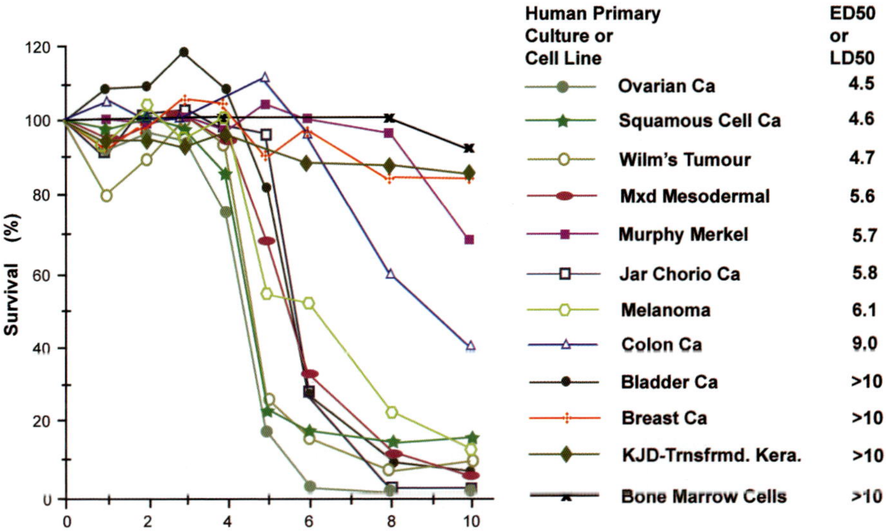

Fig. 4-3: Effect of BEC on various primary cell lines and cell cultures. This figure shows that at a concentration of 6 ug/ml of BEC, all Ovarian cancer cells are killed but no Bone Marrow cells are effected.

In Vivo studies of BEC with terminal tumours in mice, rats and large animals (horses) clearly established that BEC cured terminal tumours in animals.

The safety of BEC administration was also shown [15, 19, 28-36].

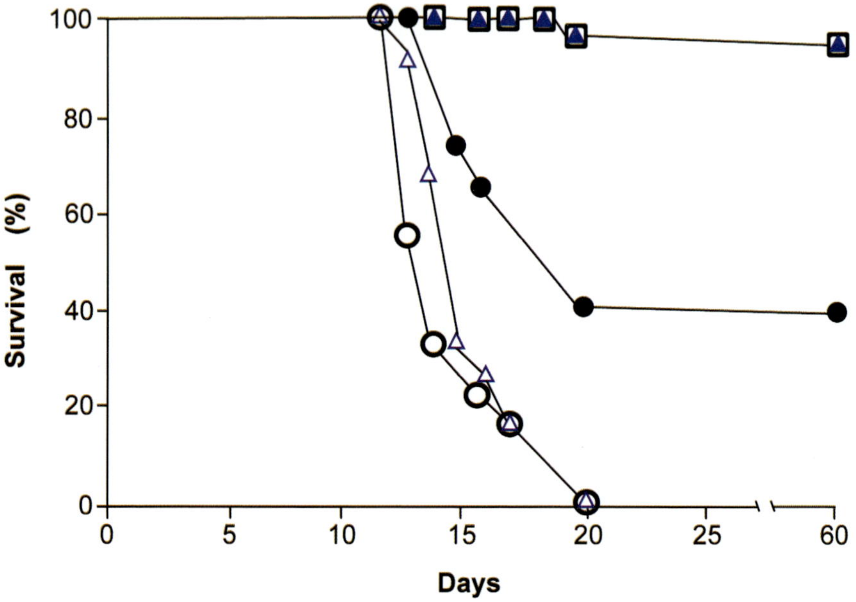

Survival of mice with Sarcoma 180 treated with varying doses of 8 mg BEC 01/kg.

–○–, control; –△–, 1 dose;–●–, 2 doses;–□–, 3 doses; –▲–, 4 doses; n = 12/group.

Fig. 4-4: This shows that two doses of BEC cured 42% whereas three and four doses cured 92% of the mice that originally had terminal cancer. All untreated mice with the cancer died at day 20.

PHASE I CLINICAL TRIALS

Here we have to distinguish between the topical application (cream) as opposed to internal use such as oral or intravenous administration. Phase I clinical trials tested BEC for safety (adverse effects) dosage tolerance, metabolism, excretion and pharmacodynamics in a small group of subjects.

BEC, at various concentrations up to 50% in a cream formulation, was shown to be very safe [15, 17-20, 37-43]. BEC when used as Curaderm BEC5 for treating non melanoma skin cancers could not be detected in the blood when analyzed for, by a very sensitive procedure, using GCMS.

So, when Curaderm BEC5 is used, no systemic absorption occurs, this is not surprising since Curaderm BEC5 contains much less BEC than is found in the eggplant. Hence, Curaderm BEC5 is extremely safe regarding BEC content! BEC when used in our studies in cream formulations established that these preparations were well tolerated and safe. Analyses of blood and urine samples during treatment with Curaderm BEC5 showed no side effects [15, 17-20, 37-43].

Haematological (Table 4-1), biochemical (Table 4-2) and urinalytical parameters obtained from 62 patients prior to, during and after Curaderm BEC5 treatment indicated that the parameters remained within the population normal range.

Table 4-1: Blood Haematological constituents monitored before, during and after Curaderm BEC5 treatment.

White blood cells	Red cell distribution width
Red blood cells	Platelet count
Haemoglobin	Mean platelet volume
Haematocrit	Heterophils
Mean corpuscular volume	Lymphocytes
Mean corpuscular haemoglobin concentration	Basophils
Mean corpuscular haemoglobin	Monocytes

There were no significant differences between before, during and after treatment in any of these parameters.

Table 4-2: Plasma Biochemical constituents monitored before, during and after Curaderm BEC5 treatment.

Sodium ion
Potassium ion
Chloride ion
Total CO2
Creatinine
Uric Acid
Urea nitrogen
Inorganic phosphate
Calcium
LDH
AST
GGT
ALT
AP
Glucose
Globulins
Albumin
Total Protein

There were no significant differences between before, during and after treatment in any of these parameters.

It was established that when a 1:1 mixture of solasonine and solamargine (the major components of BEC) was administered intravenously at a dose of 1.5 mg/kg/day over 4 hours the analyses of the pharmacokinetic data revealed that the biological half-life of solasonine was 5.57 ± 1.27 h and for solamargine this was 8.4 ± 2h. The clearance was 5.6 ± 1.6 L/h for solasonine and 3.0 ± 0.7 L/h for solamargine [44].

Unlike many other new drugs that meet the market place, we have established the mode of action of BEC. That is, we know how and why BEC selectively kills cancer cells but not normal cells. We have established that cell death occurs by apoptosis. Very interestingly, cancer cell death caused by BEC occurs while the cancer cells are "resting" and while they are "dividing". This observation is in stark contrast to the other anticancer drugs that only kill cancer cells while they are dividing, they also kill normal cells when they too are dividing.

Mechanism of Action of BEC is Unique

We have now established that cancer cell death through interaction with BEC involves a biochemical process not exploited by the industry at the time.

Unlike established anticancer drugs, BEC is not anti-mitotic in its action. That is, it does not merely interfere with the cell division process. Rather the cell itself is killed through the interaction. Importantly, the mechanism of action incorporates cell lysis through disruption of the membrane of the lysosome thus releasing the contents of the lysosome within the cell which then kills the cell through a system similar to apoptosis.

Unlike other specific anticancer treatment such as matrix metalloproteinase inhibitors, BEC is toxic to cancer cells and the tumours are eradicated as opposed to merely being constrained. Unlike anti-angiogenics, cell death from BEC is rapid and not dependent upon "starving" the cancer cell.

Apart from the obvious advantage of providing a different "line of attack" against cancer (and the concomitant implications for multi-drug resistance), we have shown and now confirmed by independent other investigators, that BEC acts preferentially upon differentiated cells (cells transformed to cancer).

This may be compared to traditional "untargeted" cytotoxics (anticancer drugs) which equally affect normal cells, resulting in severe toxic reactions in fast growing tissues and associated adverse reactions such as nausea, infection (as a result of bone marrow suppression), hair loss, severe skin reaction and ulceration.

Importantly, traditional antineoplastic (anticancer drugs) are only effective at proliferating stages of cancer growth (when the cancer cells are dividing) whereas, BEC is effective at both proliferating and resting (non dividing) cancer cells.

Pharmacodynamic studies have determined that cancer cells have a specific receptor that recognizes and binds BEC. Normal cells do not have this receptor, or if so, in only minor quantities. So BEC does not attach itself significantly to normal cells.

BEC is then internalized into the cancer cells and kills the cancer cells as shown in figures 4-5 and 4-6. The receptor on the cancer cells have been characterized as a cell membrane glycoprotein [16, 18, 20-30, 34, 45-47].

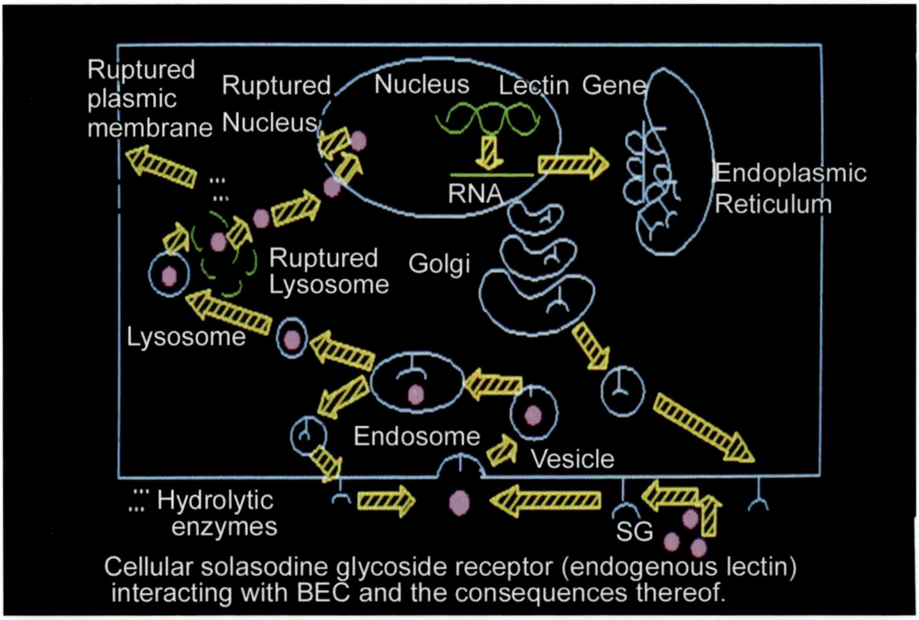

Fig. 4-5: The results of cell culture and whole animal studies indicate that the mechanism of action of BEC involves the specific recognition of the sugar parts (in particular the sugar rhamnose) of the glycoalkaloids by specific receptors, lectins, located in the plasma membrane. Binding to these receptors, forming a complex of receptor-BEC results in endocytosis of the complex. Once inside the cell, the complex is taken up by the lysosomes (stomach of cell). The lysosome breaks up BEC and the alkaloid Solasodine is generated. Solasodine in turn causes the lysosome to rupture. The contents of the lysosome is spilt into the cell. The contents of the lysosome consists of many hydrolytic enzymes that can digest fats, proteins and carbohydrates. These enzymes then break down and digest the contents of the living cell which leads to sudden death of these affected cells. Malignant cells have greater abundance of these sugar receptors (lectins) than normal cells resulting in killing of cancer cells relative to normal cells.

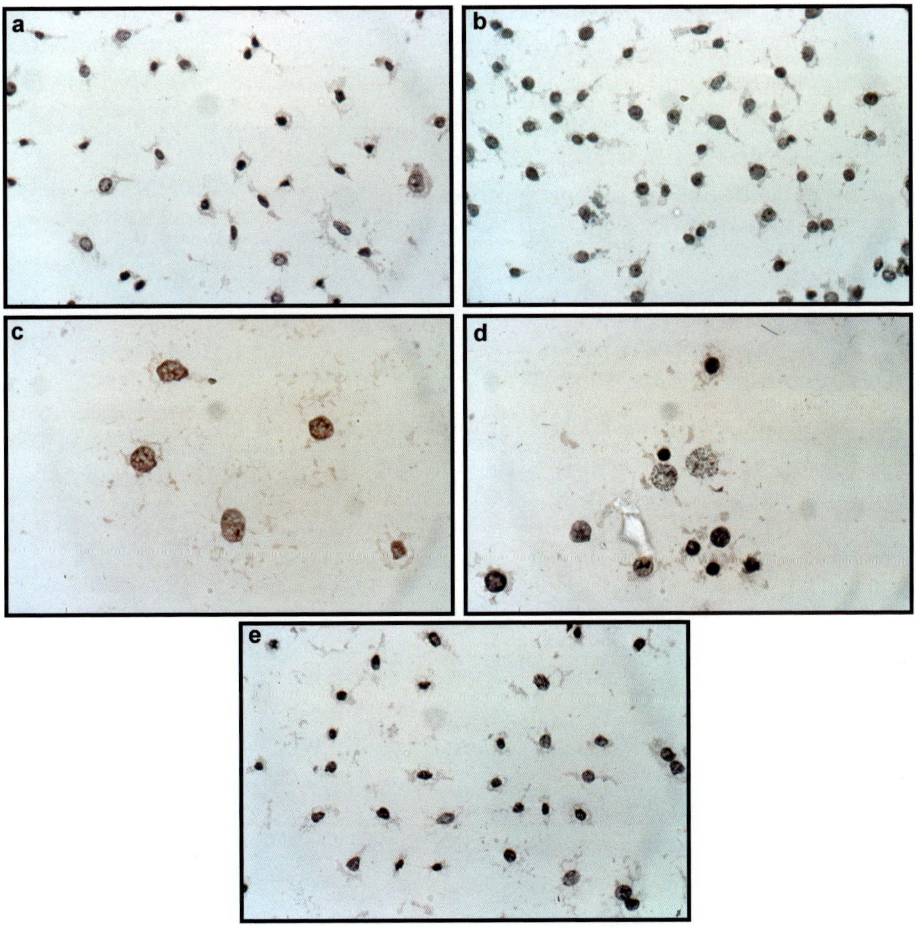

Fig. 4-6: The glycoalkaloids causes the cytoplasm of the cancer cells to undergo dissolution, the nuclei contract and become dark staining (a), nuclei then enlarge (b), the chromatin (contents of nucleus) clumps (c), and finally the nuclei disintegrate (d). Only cellular debris is left after the interaction of the cancer cells with BEC (e). This cell death is characteristic of apoptosis which is also known as programmed cancer cell death.

An analogy of the unique mechanism of action of BEC is herewith explained in simple English.

The BEC components are joined together as a sugar (glyco) part with an alkaloid (solasodine) part. Imagine that cells are represented by rooms with doors containing particular locks. A cancer cell is a room with a specific door lock which is different than the door lock that is on the normal (cell) room. The sugar (rhamnose) part of BEC may be considered as a specific key and the alkaloid is a bomb. The key of BEC only fits the lock and can open and enter the cancer cells. The key of BEC does not fit and cannot unlock the door and thus can not open or enter the normal cells. Once BEC has entered the cancer cell, something in the cell causes the bomb (solasodine alkaloid) to explode and the cancer cell is immediately killed. Because the bomb does not get into the normal cells it cannot do harm to these cells.

Thus the uniqueness of BEC as opposed to all other anti-cancer drugs is that BEC specifically only kills cancer cells without harming normal cells!

PHASE II CLINICAL TRIALS

A Phase II study marks the beginning of clinical trials on a specific, statistically determined number of patients to:

- determine the efficacy of the compound for specific indications,
- determine dosage tolerance and optimal dosage for future trials and
- identify possible adverse effects and safety risks.

SPECIFIC INDICATIONS STUDIED

Precancer
    Actinic Keratosis

Malignant Skin Cancer
    Basal Cell Carcinoma (BCC)
    Squamous Cell Carcinoma (SCC)

RESULTS OF PHASE II CLINICAL TRIALS WITH BEC

In all the clinical studies biopsies were taken before and after treatment with BEC formulations. This was done to ensure, not only clinically, but also histologically (microscopicaly) what skin cancer was treated, and to determine the effectiveness of BEC after the treatment was completed. On some occasions biopsies were taken during BEC therapy to determine by what methods BEC was killing the cancer cells.

The results of the Phase II clinical studies with 129 patients revealed that BEC in cream formulations was very effective for the chosen specific indications AK, BCC and SCC.

Patients tolerated high doses of BEC and it was determined that very low doses of BEC in the presence of keratolytic agents were optimal for treating the non melanoma skin cancers.

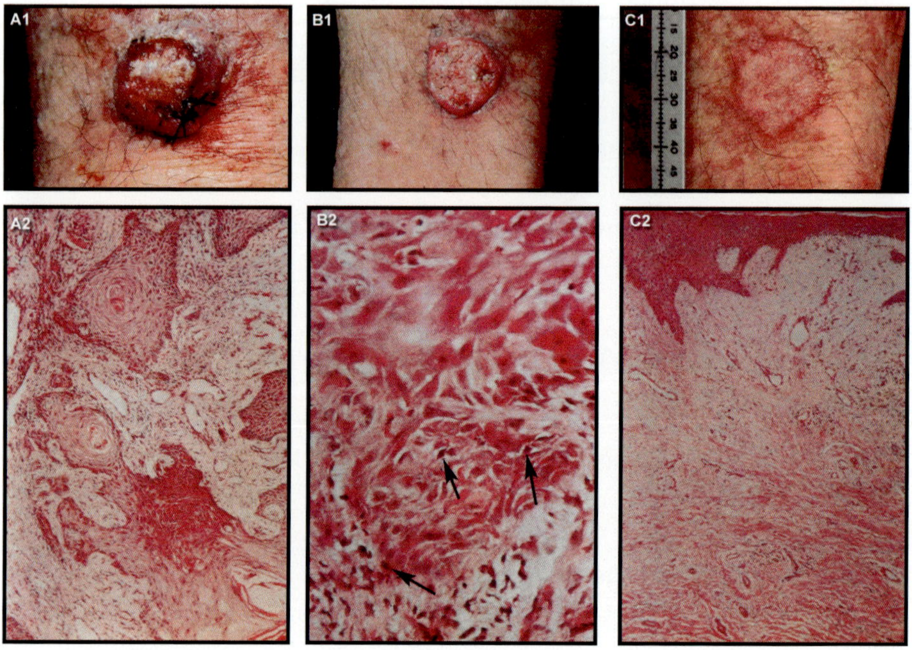

Fig. 4-7: Clinical and histological diagnosis of an SCC on a leg of a patient before treatment (lane A); during therapy (lane B); and site of treated SCC after completion of therapy (lane C). 1. clinical diagnosis; 2. histological diagnosis. Arrows indicate cancer cells dying during Curaderm BEC5 treatment (lane B; 2). The observation of this type of cell death caused by Curaderm BEC5 is similar to those obtained in cell culture studies.

The systemic adverse effects were non existent when blood chemistry, haematology and urine analysis were tested and compared before, during and after BEC therapy. No safety risks could be identified.

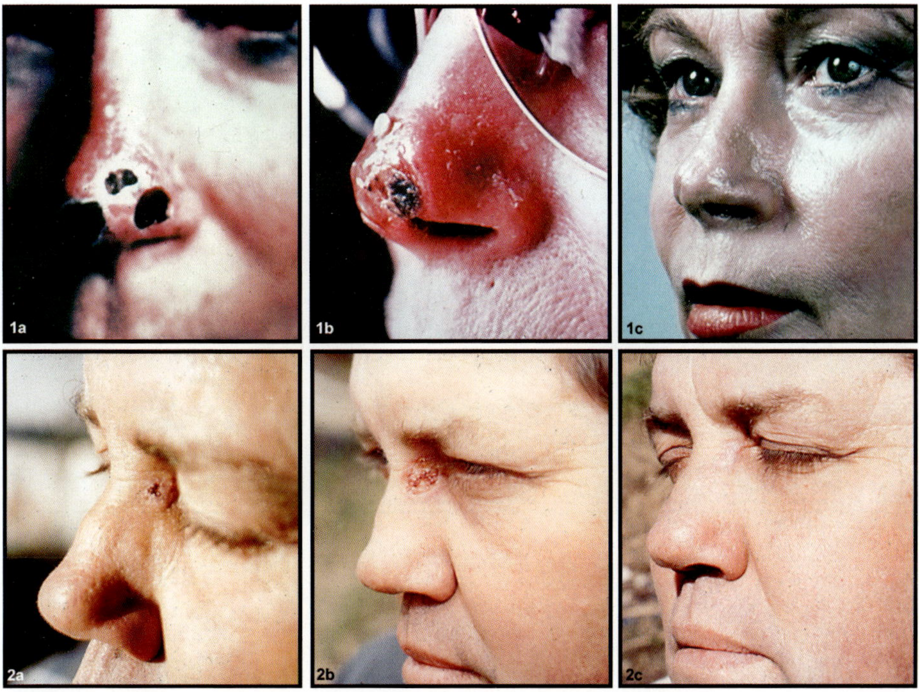

Fig. 4-8: Clinical diagnosis of a BCC on the nose of a patient before treatment with Curaderm BEC5 (1a), during therapy (1b) and site of treated BCC after completion of therapy (1c). Clinical progress of a BCC close to the eye of the patient before treatment (2a), during therapy (2b), and site of treated BCC after completion of therapy with Curaderm BEC5 (2c).

Local adverse effects were limited to local skin irritation and erythema (reddening of the skin). Some patients experienced some pain at the site of application for a short duration [15, 17-20,37-43].

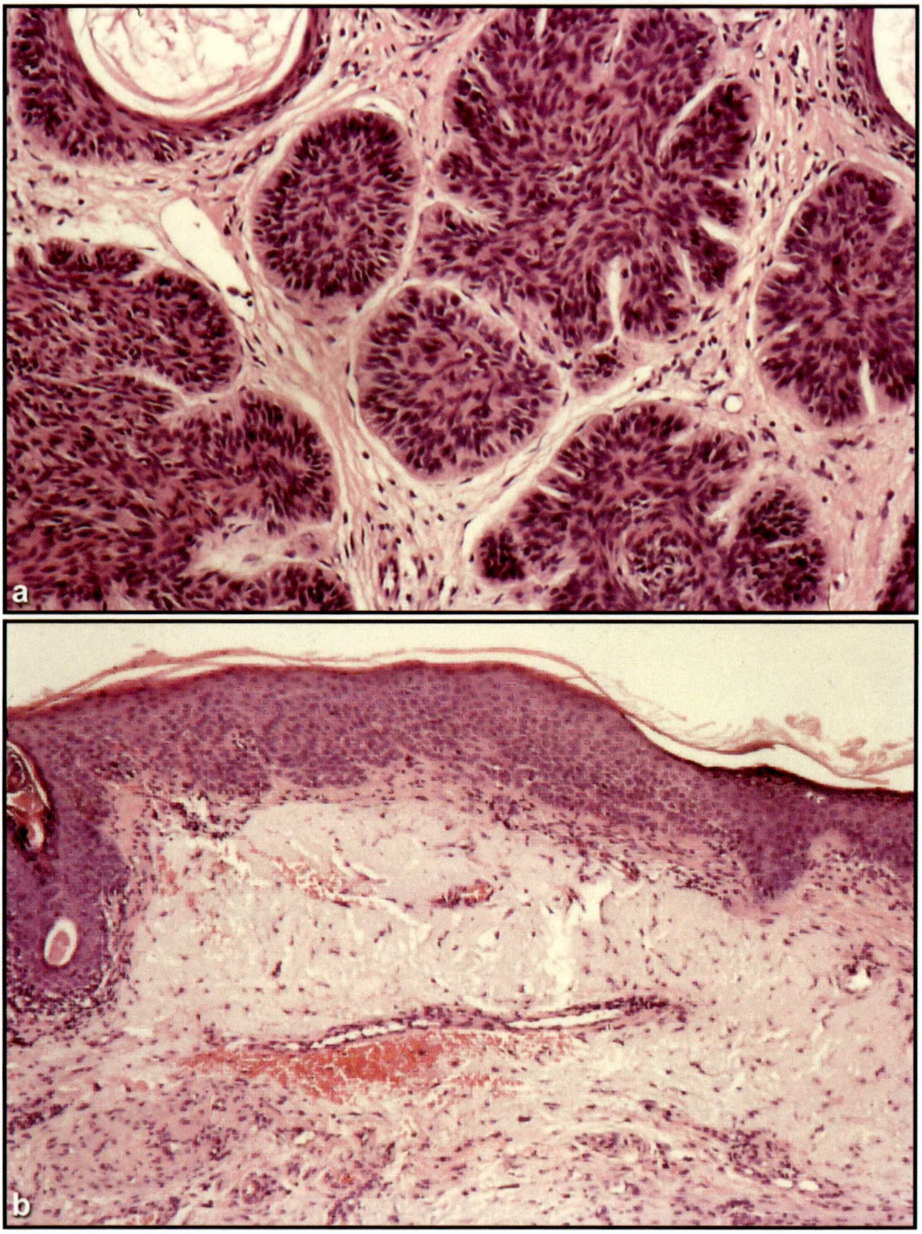

Fig. 4-9: Histological analysis of a BCC before Curaderm BEC5 therapy showing the deep infiltrated cancer cells well within the dermis (a); after Curaderm BEC5 therapy no cancer cells are present (b).

PHASE III CLINICAL TRIALS

The results of Phase III trials determined that BEC in cream formulations were effective and the safety profile was very acceptable.

Curaderm BEC5 and Phase III Clinical Studies (232 patients)

BEC was now ready to undergo a more extensive clinical trial. Curaderm BEC5 was chosen for the Phase III trials. Single and randomized double-blind placebo controlled studies were done on patients with lesions as described with the Phase II studies. A placebo is an inactive cream (in our case the same cream formulation but without the BEC) that has no treatment value. Experimental treatments are compared with placebos to assess the experimental treatment's effectiveness. The Phase III studies were done in Australia and independent multi-centre hospitals in the United Kingdom. Before the clinical studies commenced appropriate protocols were assessed to determine the appropriate execution of the clinical trials. In the United Kingdom the protocol was approved by the Medical Control Agency (MCA) for the multi-centre studies. A protocol is a carefully designed study plan to safeguard the health of the participants as well as answer specific research questions.

The results of the Phase III trials determined that Curaderm BEC5 produced success rates of 78% when Curaderm BEC5 was applied twice daily under occlusive dressing for 8 weeks. If the treatment regime was extended to 12 weeks the success rates were virtually 100%. Only local skin irritation and erythema were observed as adverse reactions. Therefore the treatment with Curaderm BEC5 was considered to be a safe therapy.

Success was defined as zero presence of non melanoma skin cancers after histological examination of samples extracted from the lesion site by punch biopsy. In addition, treated patients were followed up for over 5 years post treatment and it was determined that there were no recurrences of the treated lesions! [18-20, 41-43, 48-53] Figures 4-7 to 4-11 show cases which have been followed up 5 years post treatment.

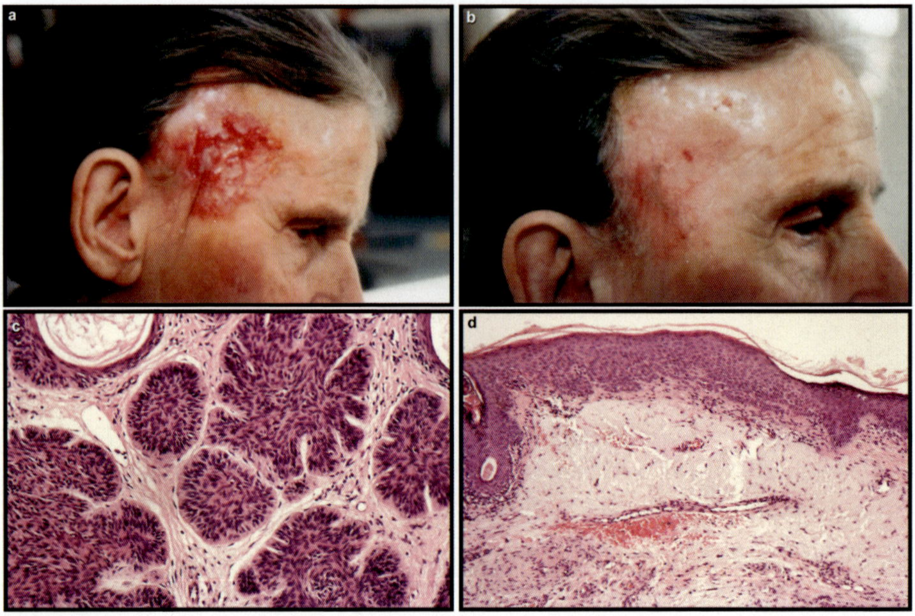

Fig. 4-10: Large BCC on the temple of a woman (a). This BCC had been surgically removed and skin grafts applied on two previous occasions only to return. Four weeks treatment with Curaderm resulted in full regression (b). Note the cosmetic result. The clinical diagnosis was confirmed histologically by punch biopsy (c). After completion of the therapy histopathology determined that no residual cancer was present (d). Clinical assessment 5 years post treatment revealed that there was no recurrence.

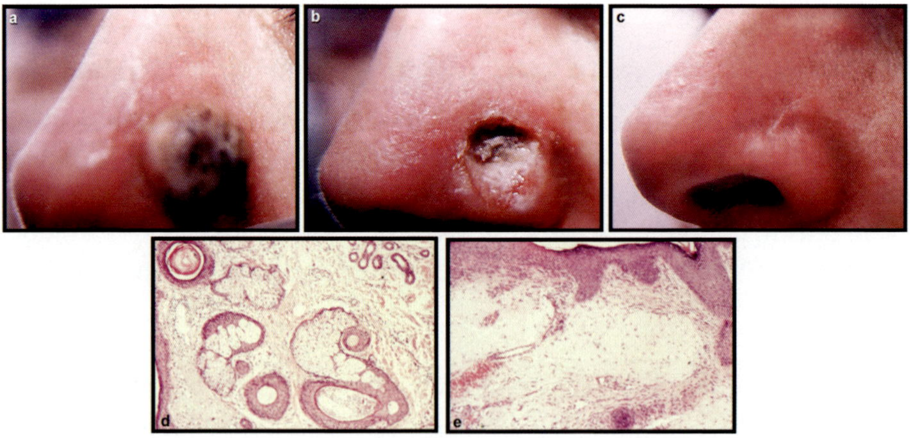

Fig. 4-11: SCC on the nose of a patient before (a), during (b) and after Curaderm treatment (c). Curaderm was applied for 5 weeks. Note the depth of the cancer as cartilage was exposed during treatment. The clinical diagnosis was confirmed histologically by punch biopsy (d). After completion of the therapy histopathology determined that no residual cancer was present (e). Clinical assessment 5 years post treatment revealed that there was no recurrence.

PHASE IV OR POST-MARKETING STUDIES

These studies are done to further confirm and describe clinical benefit of Curaderm BEC5 and yield additional information including risks and optimal use. Post-launch safety surveillance is designed to detect any rare or long-term adverse effects over a much larger patient population and timescale than was possible during the initial clinical trials.

Phase IV trials are important as they detect any rare or long-term adverse effects. Such adverse effects have resulted in the withdrawal or restriction of a drug, recent examples include cerivastatin (Baycol, Lipobay), troglithzone (Rezulin) and rofecobix (Vioxx).

Registration of adverse effects when 50,000 patients had used Curaderm BEC5 resulted in only two adverse effects documented over a ten year period with the Therapeutic Goods Administration (TGA) in Australia. Both documented adverse effects were dermatitis at the site of Curaderm BEC5 application. Cessation of Curaderm BEC5 application resulted in remission of the dermatitis. These observations secure Curaderm BEC5 treatments as having an exceptional safety profile [50, 54].

Following are some patient cases (figures 4-12 and 4-13) that have been treated with Curaderm BEC5 at the Phase IV clinical stages.

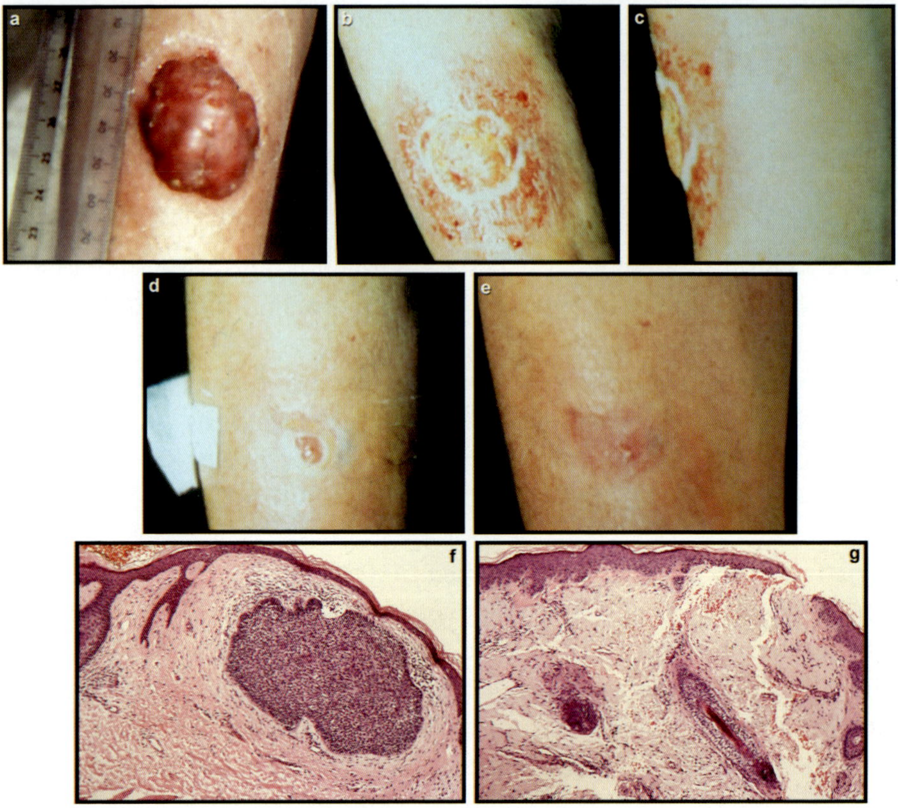

Fig. 4-12: Large BCC on the leg (a). Note how rapid the cancer was being destroyed by Curaderm during treatment (b - d) and how rapid the wound healed after 5 weeks of Curaderm therapy (e). The clinical diagnosis was confirmed histologically by punch biopsy (f). After completion of the therapy histopathology determined that no residual cancer was present (g). Clinical assessment 5 years post treatment revealed that there was no recurrence.

It can therefore be concluded that Curaderm BEC5 has been critically evaluated, and when compared to many drugs that are currently marketed, is far superior in safety and efficacy.

Curaderm BEC5 has met all the requirements regarding, research, preclinical, and clinical studies to enable its rightful place acceptance by health professionals and public as an excellent treatment for non melanoma skin cancers.

Curaderm BEC5 is the treatment of choice for non melanoma skin cancers.

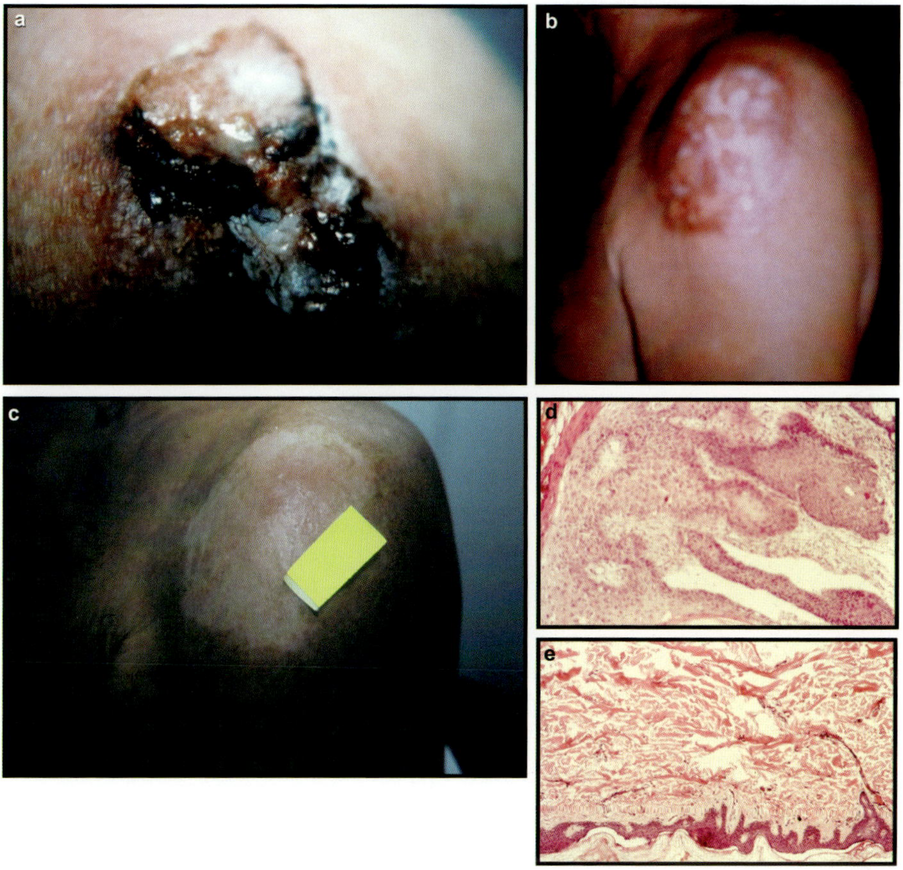

Fig. 4-13: A large SCC (approximately 8cm x 6cm) on the shoulder of a patient before (a), during (b) and after (c) treatment with Curaderm. After 10 weeks the tumour was completely healed. The clinical diagnosis was confirmed histologically by punch biopsy (d). After completion of the therapy histopathology determined that no residual cancer was present (e). Clinical assessment 5 years post treatment revealed that there was no recurrence.

Chapter 5

COMPARATIVE AVAILABLE TREATMENT REGIMES VS. CURADERM BEC5

Various forms of Surgery vs. Curaderm BEC5

BCCs can be difficult to eliminate by other widely used procedures and 5 to 10 percent of BCCs can be resistant to treatment or locally aggressive, damaging the skin around them, and sometimes invading bone and cartilage. SCCs are more difficult to treat than BCCs and like BCCs, can cause disfigurement. A small proportion (3-5 percent) can spread to distant organs and become life-threatening.

Surgery is the most common treatment for these non-melanoma skin cancers. Unfortunately recurrence rates when surgical methods are used are very high (30-67 percent) for non-melanoma skin cancers[55]. Surgical excision is invasive with the attendant risks of infection and is expensive. Where surgical excision is adopted, reconstructive surgery may also be required to address residual scarring.

Tens of thousands of patients have now used Curaderm BEC5 successfully. Most patients have treated small to medium sized skin cancers. It has already been shown in Chapter 4 that large skin cancers can also be treated with Curaderm BEC5. In this Chapter it is now shown further that not only large, but also difficult to treat areas with skin cancers are also treated effectively with Curaderm BEC5. Surgical procedures for these skin cancers would have most likely resulted in disfigurement, skin grafting and other reconstructive surgery with the likelihood of loss of parts of the body. Figures 5-1 to 5-14 show clearly that skin cancers which are either large, invasive or positioned in areas where surgery or any other treatment procedures would have resulted in highly compromising results. The results with Curaderm BEC5, as can be seen, are exceptional. In particular one case is shown whereby the patient is an own internal control, meaning that the difference between Curaderm BEC5 therapy and surgery are directly comparable. This patient who was treated with Curaderm BEC5 for an SCC on the head visited his dermatologist after Curaderm BEC5 treatment because he had bumped his head accidentally. During the consultation his dermatologist questioned the patient's participation in a Curaderm study and convinced the patient that Curaderm was unproven and that surgery was now necessary involving a skin graft on the Curaderm treated site. The patient was intimidated and scared and agreed to the surgery but requested the histological evidence after surgery that the SCC was still present following Curaderm therapy. After the surgery was completed, six areas of the surgically removed tissue representing the entire area of the surgically excised skin were analyzed histologically. There were no traces of cancer whatsoever in the surgically removed tissue. Thus, Curaderm had already removed the cancer altogether. Table 5-1 shows the histopathological report of the large surgically removed tissue. No traces of cancer could be found. This is a unique case, because it shows the end result of surgery and skin graft (Fig. 5-15) albeit from a suspected SCC lesion (already successfully removed by Curaderm BEC5 therapy) and the end result of the Curaderm BEC5 successful treatment (Figure 5-12) of the true lesion on the same patient at the same lesion site. These observations have now been published in a scientific journal [56]. This is truly a case of Surgery vs. Curaderm BEC5. Thus, it can be concluded that Curaderm BEC5 is advantageous over surgical excision by demonstrating largely scar-free healing and complete removal of the cancer cells. Curaderm BEC5 treatment is efficacious convenient and inexpensive, being a patient administered therapy with excellent cosmetic results.

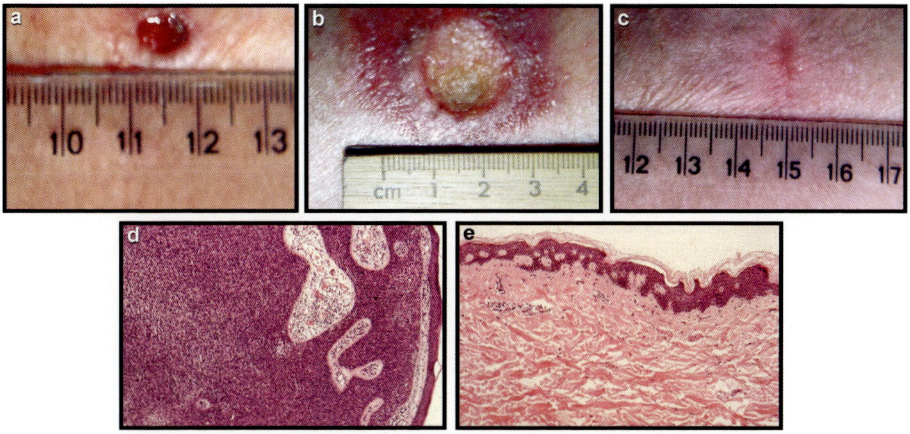

Fig. 5-1: BCC on the arm. Note initially how small the lesion appeared before Curaderm therapy (a). During therapy it is clear that Curaderm was attacking and killing all the cancerous cells (b), which prior to Curaderm treatment were not apparent. Curaderm exposes the clinically unnoticed cancer cells and eliminates them (c). Treatment period for this patient was 8 weeks. The clinical diagnosis was confirmed histologically by punch biopsy (d). After completion of the therapy histopathology determined that no residual cancer was present (e). Clinical assessment 5 years post treatment revealed that there was no recurrence.

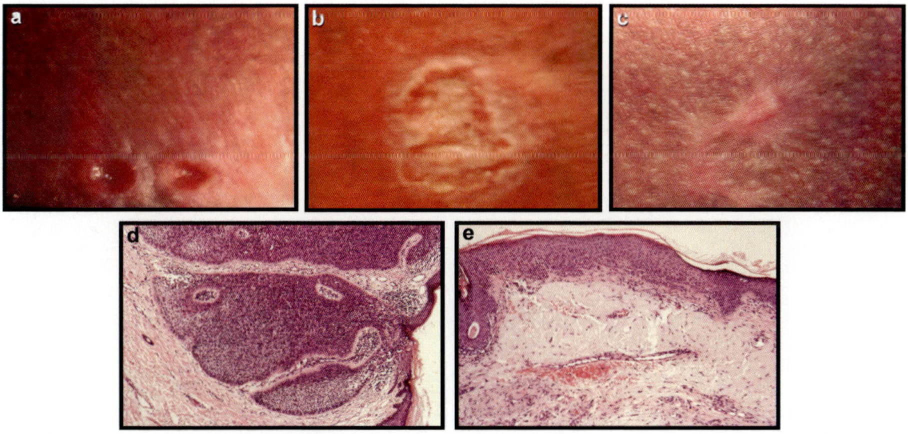

Fig. 5-2: A clinically diagnosed BCC before treatment which appears to be two distinct lesions (a). During treatment Curaderm shows that it is one large BCC (3cm x 4cm) (b). After treatment the lesion is completely ablated and some scar tissue can be seen (c). Treatment period was 16 weeks. Histological analysis before Curaderm therapy shows characteristic infiltrated cancer cells well within the dermis (d); after Curaderm therapy there are no cancer cells (e). Clinical assessment 5 years post treatment revealed that there was no recurrence.

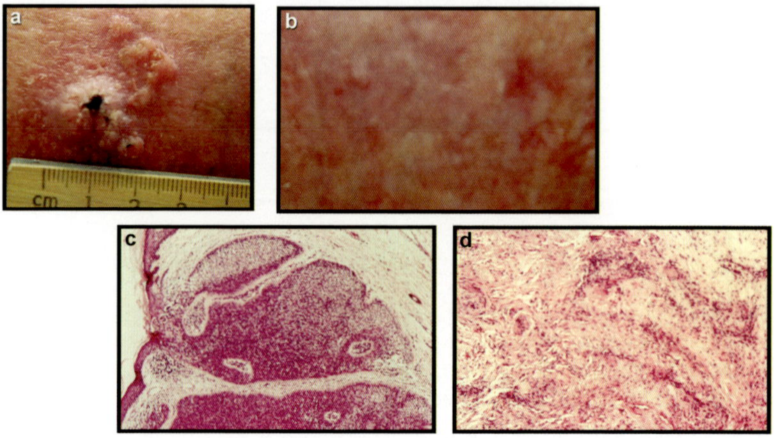

Fig. 5-3: BCC before treatment (a) and after 8 weeks of Curaderm treatment (b). The clinical diagnosis was confirmed histologically by punch biopsy (c). After completion of the therapy histopathology determined that no residual cancer was present (d). Clinical assessment 5 years post treatment revealed that there was no recurrence.

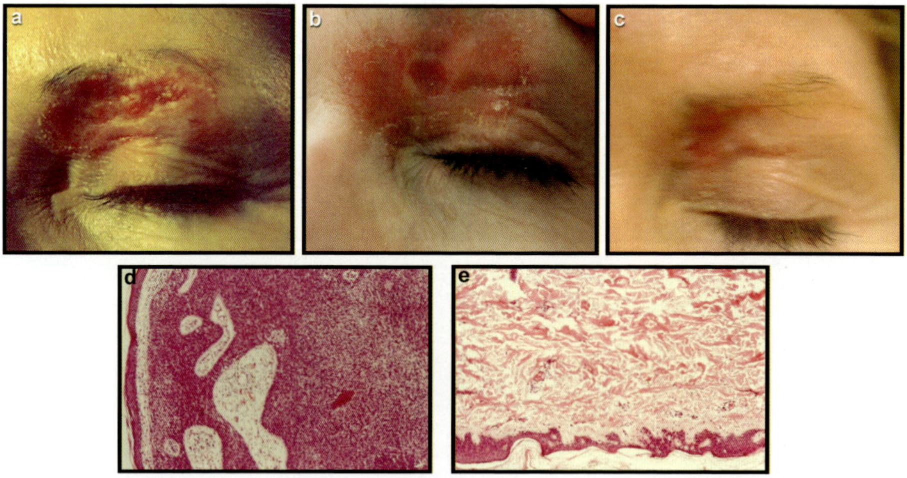

Fig. 5-4: BCC over the left eye of a patient before (a), during (b) and after Curaderm treatment (c). Careful application of Curaderm was required to ensure that the cream did not enter the eye. During Curaderm therapy the distinct tumour can be seen surrounded by some inflammation. After treatment there was no trace of the BCC. Confirmation by histological analysis of the BCC before treatment (d) and after treatment (e) are shown. The total treatment period was 9 weeks. Clinical assessment 5 years post treatment revealed that there was no recurrence.

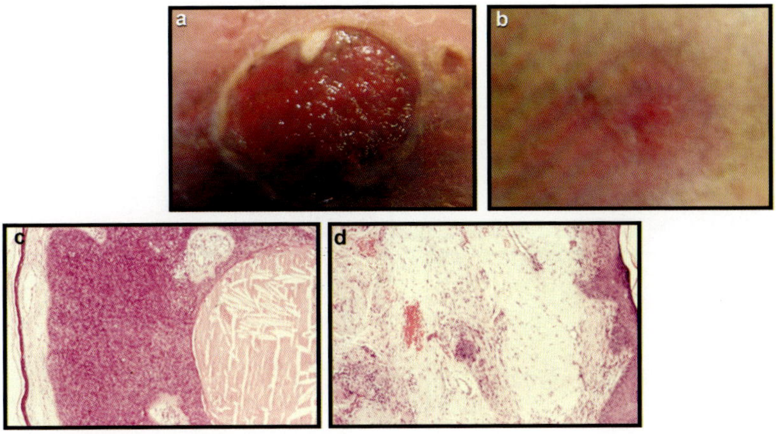

Fig. 5-5: Clinical (a) and histological (c) diagnosed BCC before Curaderm treatment. The diameter of the lesion was 5cm. Clinical (b) and histological (d) analyses after treatment. Duration of treatment was 8 weeks. Clinical assessment 5 years post treatment revealed that there was no recurrence.

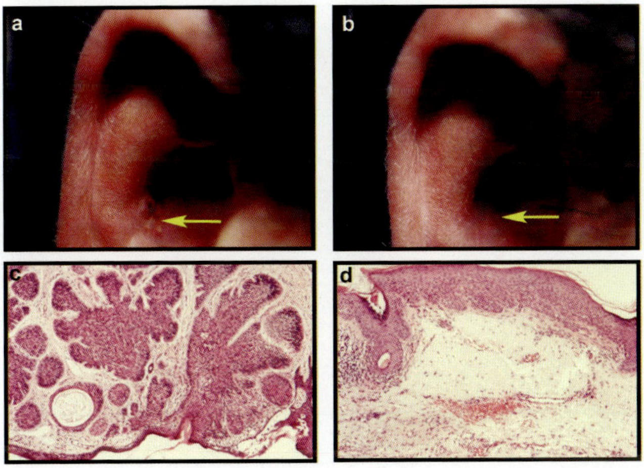

Fig. 5-6: Clinical (a) and histological (c) diagnosed BCC in the ear of a patient before Curaderm treatment. Clinical (b) and histological (d) analyses after treatment. Duration of treatment was 10 weeks. Clinical assessment 5 years post treatment revealed that there was no recurrence.

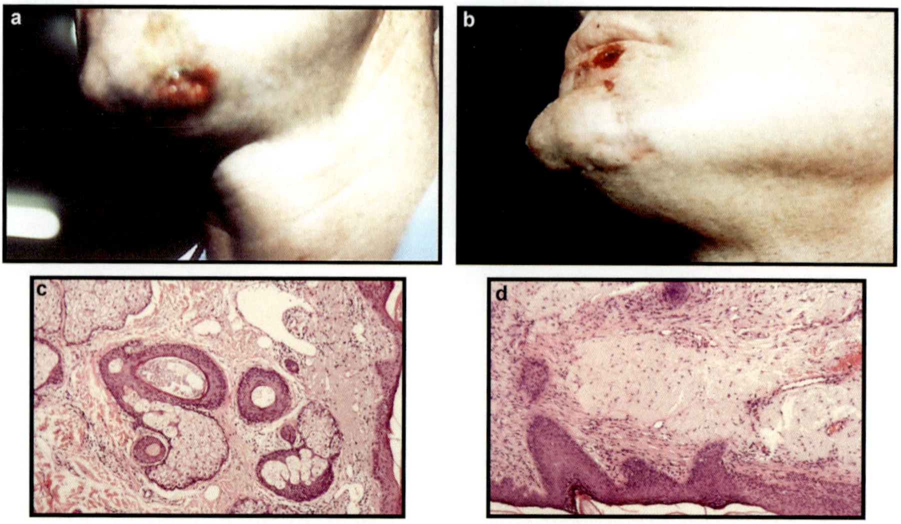

Fig. 5-7: This patient had a deep seated SCC under the chin (a). After 6 weeks treatment with Curaderm the cancer cleared up (b). The clinical diagnosis was confirmed histologically by punch biopsy (c). After completion of the therapy histopathology determined that no residual cancer was present (d). Clinical assessment 5 years post treatment revealed that there was no recurrence.

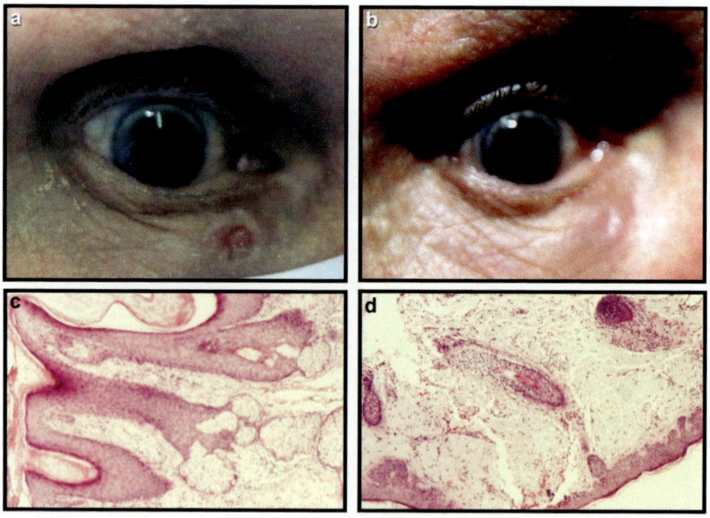

Fig. 5-8: SCC under the right eye of a patient before (a) and after Curaderm treatment (b). Careful application of Curaderm was required to ensure that the cream did not enter the eye. After treatment there was no trace of the SCC. Confirmation by histological analysis of the SCC before treatment (c) and after treatment (d) are shown. The total treatment period was 14 weeks. Clinical assessment 5 years post treatment revealed that there was no recurrence.

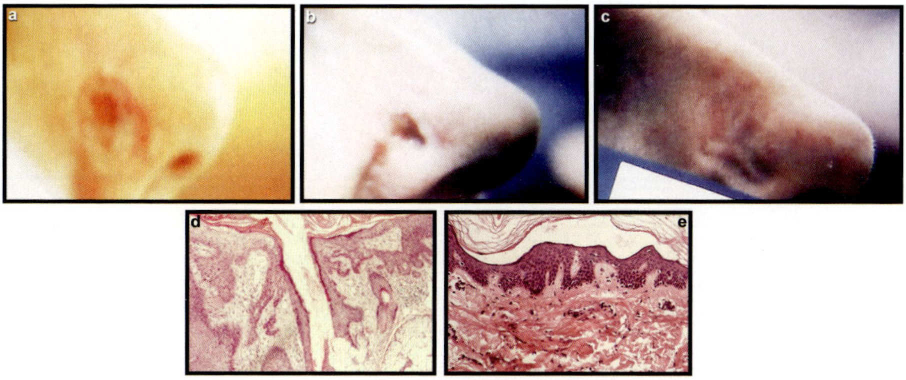

Fig. 5-9: SCC on the nose of a patient before (a), during (b) and after treatment with Curaderm (c). Treatment duration was 16 weeks. The clinical diagnosis was confirmed histologically by punch biopsy (d). After completion of the therapy histopathology determined that no residual cancer was present (e). Clinical assessment 5 years post treatment revealed that there was no recurrence.

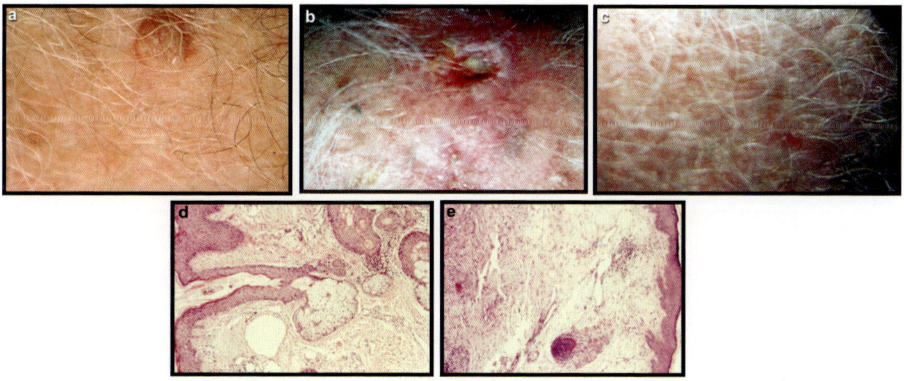

Fig. 5-10: SCC on the head of a patient before (a), during (b) and after Curaderm treatment (c). Treatment duration was 6 weeks. The clinical diagnosis was confirmed histologically by punch biopsy (d). After completion of the therapy histopathology determined that no residual cancer was present (e). Clinical assessment 5 years post treatment revealed that there was no recurrence.

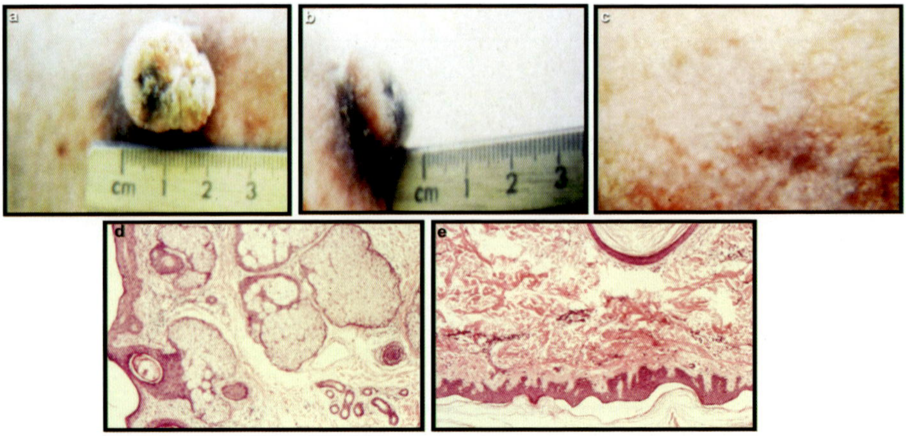

Fig. 5-11: A protruding SCC before (a, b) and after Curaderm therapy (c). Treatment duration was 8 weeks. The clinical diagnosis was confirmed histologically by punch biopsy (d). After completion of the therapy histopathology determined that no residual cancer was present (e). Clinical assessment 5 years post treatment revealed that there was no recurrence.

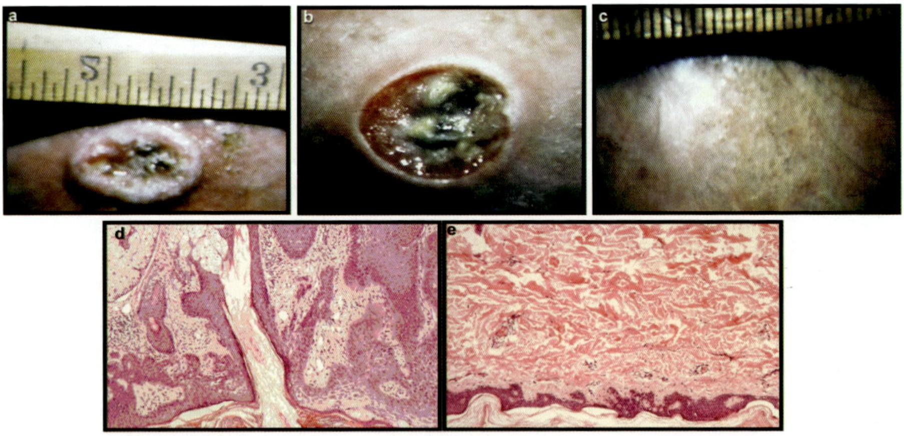

Fig. 5-12: SCC showing the effectiveness of Curaderm to specifically target cancer cells without affecting normal cells. Before Curaderm treatment (a), during Curaderm treatment (b) and after treatment (c). Treatment duration was 8 weeks. The clinical diagnosis was confirmed histologically by punch biopsy (d). After completion of the therapy histopathology determined that no residual cancer was present (e).

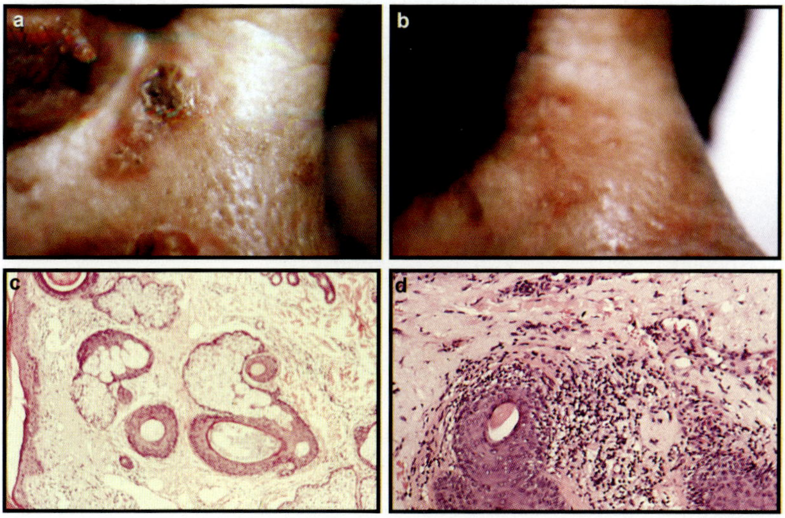

Fig. 5-13: SCC on the nose close to the eye (a). This SCC was starting to impair the vision of the patient. After Curaderm therapy the lesion was ablated (b). After completion on treatment the vision was restored. Treatment duration was 10 weeks. The clinical diagnosis was confirmed histologically by punch biopsy (c). After completion of the therapy histopathology determined that no residual cancer was present (d). Clinical assessment 5 years post treatment revealed that there was no recurrence.

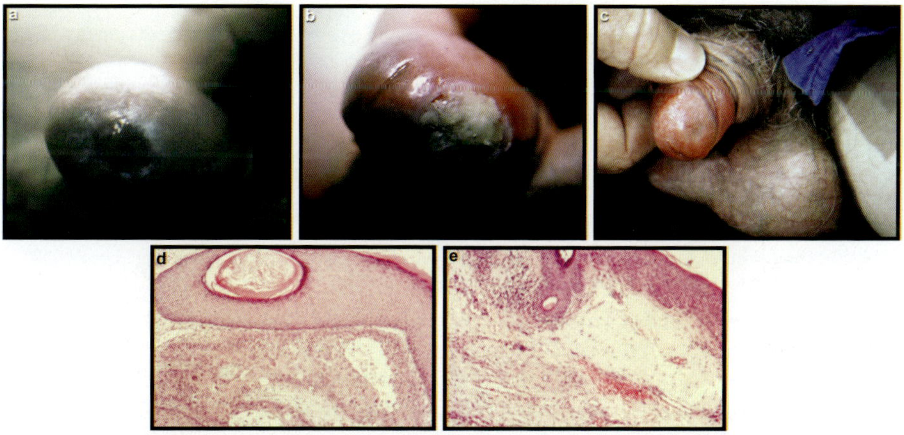

Fig. 5-14: An intra-epithelial SCC on the penis of a patient before (a), during (b) and after Curaderm therapy (c). The prognosis of this patient before treatment with Curaderm was amputation. Treatment period was 6 weeks. The clinical diagnosis was confirmed histologically by biopsy (d). After completion of the therapy histopathology determined that no residual cancer was present (e). Clinical assessment 5 years post treatment revealed that there was no recurrence.

QUEENSLAND HEALTH PATHOLOGY SERVICE – Princess Alexandra Hospital

Patient Location	**A3 – Clinics**	**UR No**	**PA813681**
Consultant	**Theile, David R. (PAH)**	**Name**	**ROBERTS**
Requesting MO	**Dr David R, Theile**	**Given Name**	**Alan Leslie Sex M**
	Princess Alexandra	**DOB**	**18-Jun-1944 Age 55 years**
	Ipswich Road	**Patient Address**	**Boundary Creek Road**
	Wooloongabba Q 4102		**Bentley NSW 2480**

Collected ??:??17-Dec-99 Lab No 1922-4391

Histopathology Report **Biopsy No:**

Macroscopic by Dr T Robertson

CLINICAL NOTES
Frozen sections SCC poorly differentiated? Lateral margin clear.

MACROSCOPIC DESCRIPTION
6 specimens received. Specimen 1 labelled "right anterior" and consists of a skin ellipse meas. 20x3x5mm. Blocked in toto block A for froz. Sect. Frozen sections diagnosis: IB/RAA no evidence of malignancy.

Specimen 2 labelled "right posterior" and consists of skin ellipse meas. 25x3x3mm. Blocked in toto block B for frozen sect. Frozen sections diagnosis: IB/RAA no evidence of malignancy.

Specimen 3 labelled "left anterior" and consists of a skin ellipse meas. 25x3x5mm. Blocked in toto block C for frozen sect. Frozen sections diagnosis: IB/RAA no evidence of malignancy.

Specimen 4 labelled "left posterior" and consists of a skin ellipse meas. 25x3x5mm. Blocked in toto block D for frozen sect. Frozen sections diagnosis: IB/RAA no evidence of malignancy.

Specimen 5 labelled "SCC scalp, long anterior, short right lateral" and consists of a tear drop shaped portion of skin meas. 85mm anterior to posterior by 45mm right to left. In the centre of the specimen is an irregular shaped elongated focally ulcerated plaque meas. 63x28mm. The specimen is inked in blue and the right lateral margin scored. Sectioning the tissue reveals poorly defined induration which appears to extend into subcutis. Summary of sects. E 3 LS to 12 o'clock; F to L 7 TS blocked from anterior to posterior; M 2 LS to 6 o'clock.

Specimen 6 labelled "skin lesion posterior scalp" and consists of an oval of skin meas. 50x42x4mm with a central poorly defined area of induration showing depression meas. 35x22mm. A marker suture is present at one point which is orientated to posterior (6 o'clock). The 12 o'clock margin is scored. Summary of secs. N-P 3 TS; Q 3 LS to 3 o'clock; R 3 LS to 9 o'clock. (bp)

MICROSCOPIC DESCRIPTION
1 to 4. Paraffin sections confirm the frozen section diagnosis and show no evidence of malignancy in any of the 4 specimens.

5. The sections show an extensive area of superficial ulceration of the skin with scale crust and intense subjacent chronic inflammation with numerous plasma cells associated with dermal scarring. Focal solar keretosis is present on the adjacent skin. There is no evidence of any malignancy in several

6. The sections show foci of superficial ulceration with scale crust and subjacent mild to moderate chronic inflammation and scarring. There is no evidence of malignancy in several sections.

SUMMARY
Non-specific chronic ulceration of skin of scalp. No evidence of malignancy.
(ra)

Dr TE Robertson, Dr RA Axelsen

Table 5-1: Histopathology report of the patient described in figures 5-12 and 5-15.

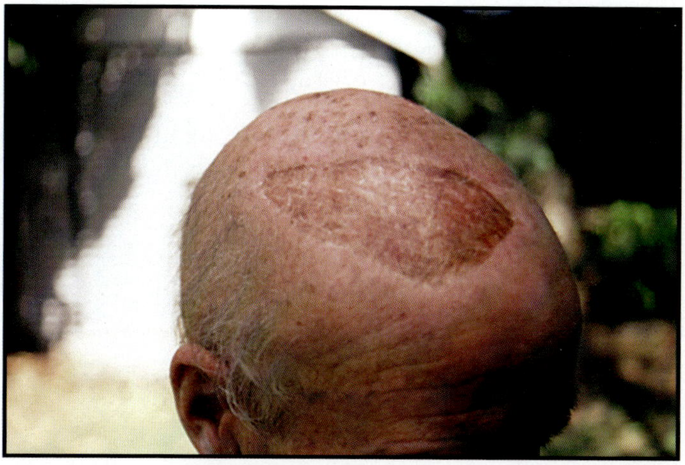

Fig. 5-15: Skin graft of a surgically removed area which the dermatologist assumed had residual cancer after Curaderm therapy. This patient is represented by Fig. 5-12. Analysis of the surgically removed area of the skin revealed that there was no residual cancer present (see Table 5-1), thus this patient underwent unnecessary surgery and skin grafting. Curaderm had already successfully removed all cancer cells prior to skin graft surgery.

5-Fluorouracil (5-FU) vs. Curaderm BEC5

Of the established treatment regimes, 5-FU has been used extensively as an alternative to surgery and cryotherapy in respect of actinic keratoses. The use of 5-FU for the treatment of superficial BCC was established after it was prescribed on an "off-label" basis. Efficacy rate of 5-FU is very low against superficial BCC. Additionally, 5-FU is a "conventional" cytotoxic compound with a corresponding inherent toxicity profile and so should be used sparingly. Consequently physicians are reluctant to prescribe 5-FU for use on BCCs that are not located on "low risk" sites such as limbs or trunk area.

By comparison, Curaderm BEC5 has an exceptional safety profile. It has been established that neither the active glycoalkaloids (BEC) ingredients of this natural drug nor their breakdown products enter the blood stream in quantities detectable by a very sensitive procedure (Mass spectrometry). Local effects of use are limited to slight inflammation, erythema (reddening of the skin) and stinging.

Moreover, Curaderm BEC5 preferentially seeks out and destroys cancer cells and can be used upon substantial and sub-cutaneous (deep within the skin) cancers, rendering it a far superior option. Contrast the position with 5-FU which does not differentiate in killing dividing cells, whether they are normal or cancerous. Curaderm BEC5 preferentially kills cancer cells only and not normal cells. In addition Curaderm BEC5 kills cancer cells whether they are dividing or whether they are "resting". Finally, Curaderm BEC5 has a clinically proven very high efficacy rate.

Photo-Dynamic Therapy (PDT) vs. Curaderm BEC5

In some authorities PDT has been approved for the treatment of BCC. PDT has significant limitations. The efficacy of PDT in the treatment of BCCs is low and is limited to superficial BCCs. Side effects can prove disproportionate to the disease and may include local swelling and inflammation in and around the oesaphagus and lungs. All PDT patients experience photosensitivity for approximately 30 days due to the continued presence of the drug in the body, and exposure to bright light or direct sunlight should be avoided to prevent sunburn, redness and swelling. Other reported side effects include nausea, fever and/or constipation. The patients are advised to avoid direct sunlight and bright indoor light for at least six weeks after treatment.

PDT centres are capital intensive and so access is limited. Moreover, not every centre incorporates a light source suitable for the treatment of all possible PDT treatable cancers. In addition, cost, lack of safety and limited efficacy are significant deterrents for PDT compared to Curaderm BEC5. For all these reasons PDT is not used much.

Imiquimod vs. Curaderm BEC5

Imiquimod (as "Aldara") is presently available as a treatment for external anogenital warts. Unlike Curaderm BEC5, topical Aldara demonstrates systemic toxicity and reported adverse drug reactions include fever and general malaise. When used to treat BCCs a range of very serious adverse effects have been reported.

Table 5-2 shows comparative profiles of the various treatment types:

Treatment Type	Cost	Efficacy	Safety	Superficial and Morphoeic	Selectivity	Cosmetic Appearance
Surgery	High	High	Moderate	Both	High	Variable
5-FU	Low	Low	Low	Superficial	None	Good
PDT	Very High	Limited	Side Effects	Superficial	High	Good
Aldara	Low	Limited	Side Effects	Superficial	Moderate	Variable
Curaderm BEC5	Low	High	High	Both	High	Very Good

Table 5-2: The above Table refers to BCCs. Only surgery and Curaderm BEC5 have proven to be effective in the treatment of SCCs.

It is important to note that the clinico-physical health benefits go hand-in-hand with mental benefits resulting in improved lifestyles. Herewith, a letter received from a patient together with photographs of before, during and after Curaderm BEC5 therapy of a large SCC on the head.

I have been a candidate for skin cancer for many years.
Some 6 years ago I was in and out of hospital with overnight stays (at least 3 times a year) having several skin cancers surgically removed each time. These skin cancers lesions were removed from my upper body, upper arms, face, head & a graft on my ear. During this time I would have had over 300 stitches, no fun I can assure you.
Many of these skin cancers lesions had been previously removed with Liquid Nitrogen but reoccurred at a later date.
As I thought it was now time for Surgery to end once and for all. How wrong was I. Not only was I left with surgical scars but the lesions reoccurred once again.
Then some 2 - 3 years ago I was introduced to a wonderful natural product called Curaderm. After investigations I found that Curaderm had been clinically proven. This cream is made from an active ingredient extract from Egg Plant.

I have been using this product ever since, it is easy to use in my own home, can carry the Curaderm in my pocket, do not have to travel vast distances for surgery, no anesthetic, no stitches to be removed and works out to be an inexpensive medication to have in my medicine chest. Curaderm has now advanced to Curaderm BEC 5. During this time my wife has treated over 50 BCCs on my head & back and a large SCC on my head. I am able to treat the rest of these lesions.
As my family has a history of skin cancers and my brother passed away due to the ignorance of skin cancer I have made myself become very aware of all types of products available for cures. Curaderm definitely comes up on the top of my list.

Please refer to photograghs. [Fig. 5-16]

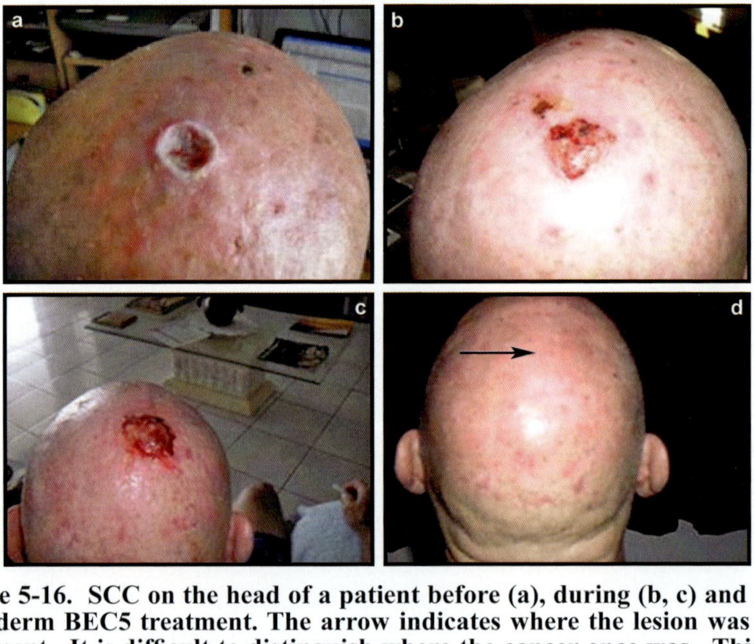

Figure 5-16. SCC on the head of a patient before (a), during (b, c) and after (d) Curaderm BEC5 treatment. The arrow indicates where the lesion was prior to treatment. It is difficult to distinguish where the cancer once was. This SCC is similar to the one described earlier (Figures 5-12, 5-15). Again it is shown that the cosmetic result is excellent.

Although Curaderm BEC5 treats large skin cancer lesions, it is extremely important that patients in consultation with their health professionals treat skin cancers in their early stages. The smaller the lesion, the shorter the treatment duration and the less troublesome for the patient.

Chapter 6

Recommended Curaderm BEC5 Treatment Procedure

Before applying Curaderm BEC5 cream, patients are instructed to wash the lesion and the surrounding area with a mild, non-irritating soap, to rinse with water, and allow the area to dry thoroughly. Curaderm BEC5 is to be applied to the lesions in sufficient quantity to cover each lesion. The cream is not to extend more than 0.5cm onto the apparently normal skin surrounding the edge of the lesion. Each lesion is to be covered with an occlusive dressing (paper tape) until the next application of Curaderm BEC5. The cream is to be applied to each lesion using the dropper lid on the plastic container by gently squeezing the container at least twice daily, ie, at least every 12 hours up until the lesion has been completely ablated and replaced with normal skin.

Patients are to wash their hands after application of Curaderm BEC5 and avoid contact of the cream with their eyes. Cosmetics are not to be used on the affected areas and patients are cautioned to avoid sun exposure.

If the dressing becomes detached before the next scheduled dosing, the patient is instructed to reapply new cream and a new dressing. The affected area is to be kept covered at all times during the treatment period.

Curaderm BEC5 is stored below 25°C and maintained under adequate security. If the cream is exposed to higher temperatures and the cream separates to a liquid form then the separated cream cannot be used further.

The patient is explained to expect that, initially during treatment, the lesion diameter will increase significantly and then as treatment progresses the diameter of the lesion will decrease until all cancer cells are replaced with normal cells.

Figure 6-1 illustrates observable lesion changes in diameter during Curaderm BEC5 therapy up to week 6 and after cessation of Curaderm BEC5 therapy. In these studies Curaderm BEC5 was stopped after 8 weeks therapy. From weeks 2 to 6, Curaderm BEC5 treatment resulted in significant increases in lesions diameter. After 6 weeks of treatment the lesion size was reduced. Follow-up studies for 6 months and 1 year show clearly that all the lesions had completely resolved. The number of patients studied here were 31 to 57. The reason of the initial increase in lesion size is the Curaderm BEC5 is seeking and destroying the cancer cells that are initially not visible to the bare eyes.

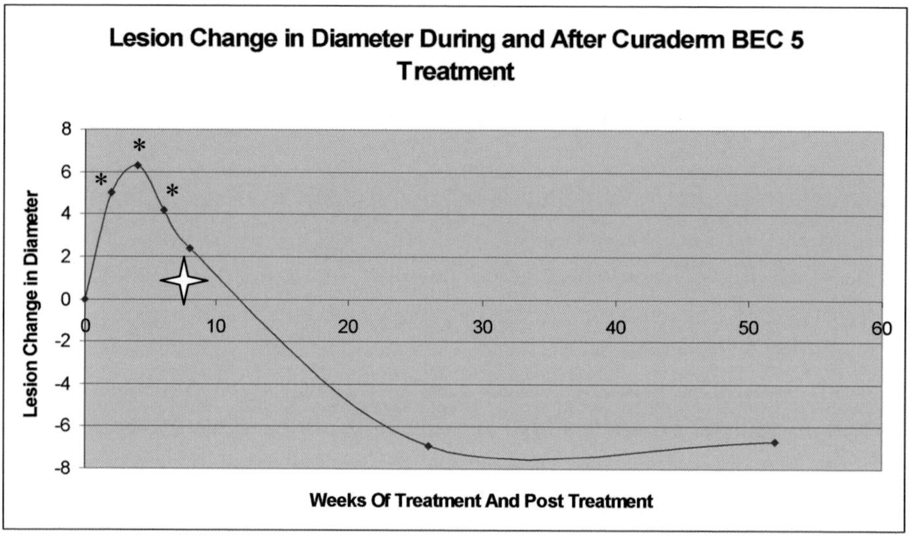

Fig. 6-1: Changes in lesion diameter during and after Curaderm BEC5 treatment.

The correlation between the diameter (mm) of the lesion and weeks of treatment with Curaderm BEC 5.

The symbol * illustrates significant differences (Mann-Whitney U-test) from the time prior to treatment.

The symbol ✧ denotes the end of Curaderm BEC 5 therapy.

Schematic Representation of the Sequential Events of Skin Cancer Treatment with Curaderm BEC5

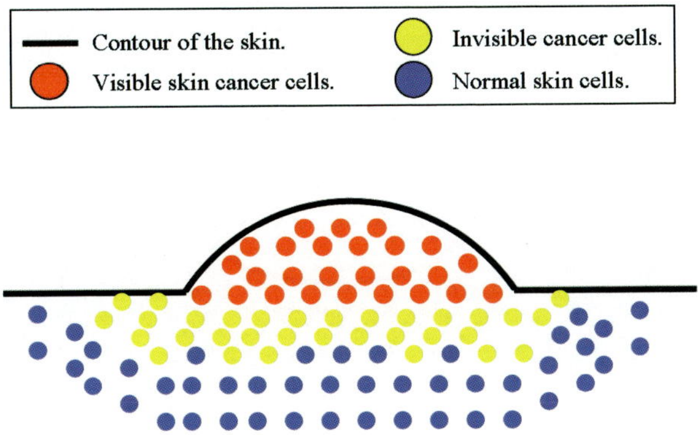

Before Curaderm BEC5 treatment.
The lesion protrudes from the skin.
Start Curaderm BEC5 treatment.

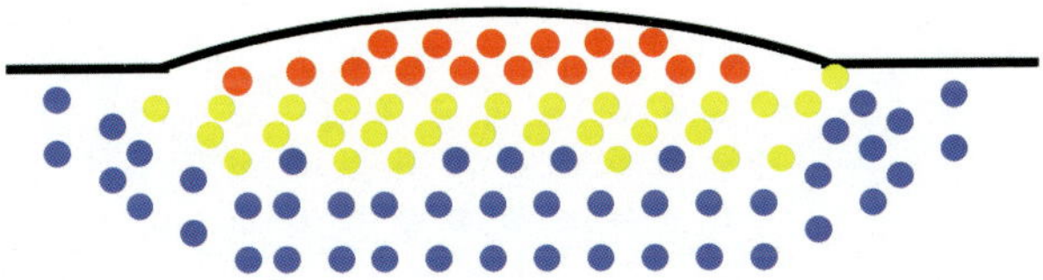

During Curaderm BEC5 treatment.
Lesion diameter is larger than before treatment. Curaderm BEC5 seeks out and destroys cancer cells well within the "apparently" normal margin and exposes and kills the "hidden" cancer cells. Continue to treat lesion with Curaderm BEC5.

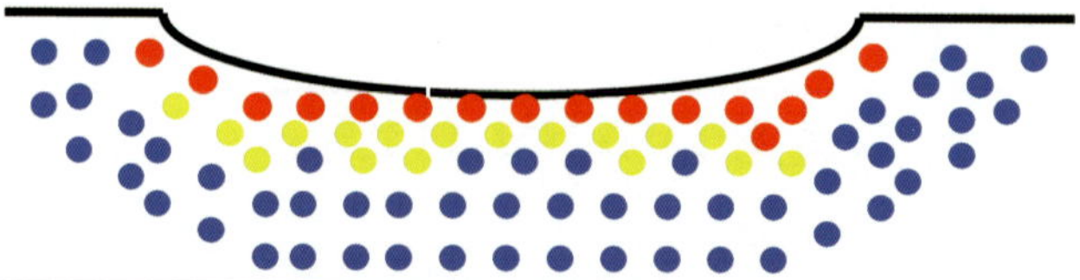

During Curaderm BEC5 treatment.
Curaderm BEC5 continues to kill the cancer cells that are well within the epidermis and dermis, causing an apparent hole in the skin. Continue to treat lesion with Curaderm BEC5.

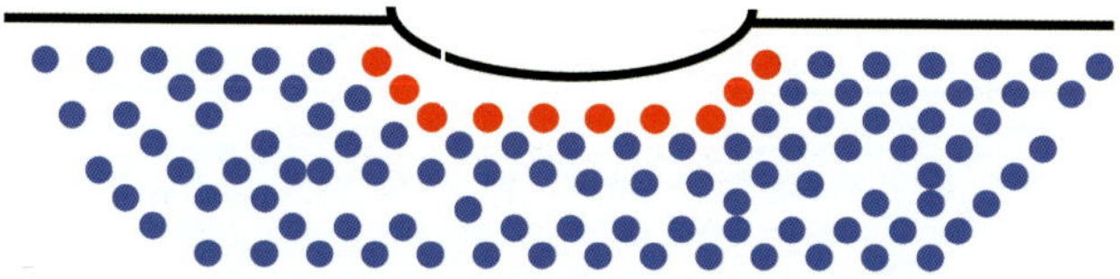

During Curaderm BEC5 treatment.
Most of the cancer cells have been killed. The killed cancer cells are replaced by normal cells. The diameter of the cancer is now smaller. Continue to treat lesion with Curaderm BEC5.

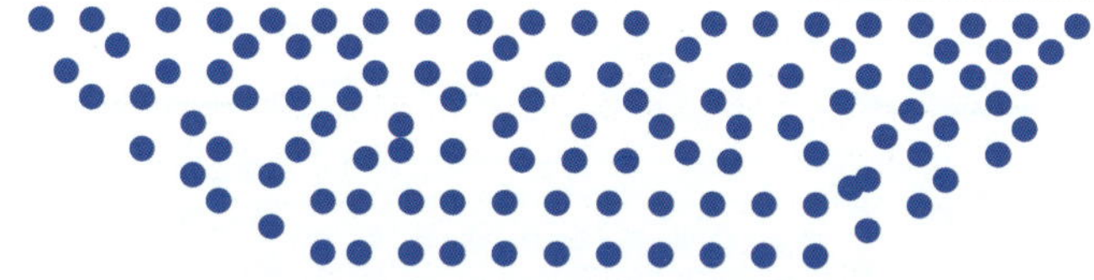

Conclusion of Curaderm BEC5 treatment.
No more cancer cells are present, only normal cells. Stop Curaderm BEC5 treatment.

Fig. 6-2: Schematic Representation of the Sequential Events of Skin Cancer Treatment with Curaderm BEC5

Clinical Representation of the Sequential Events of Skin Cancer Treatment with Curaderm BEC5

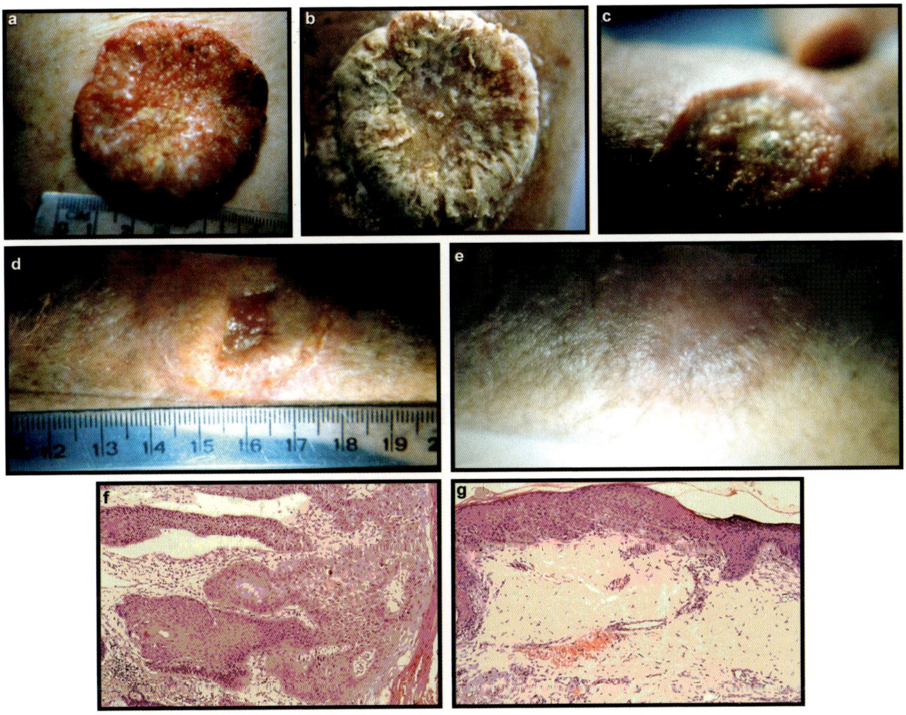

Fig. 6-3: A very large SCC, 6cm in diameter, before (a), during (b – d), and after (e) treatment with Curaderm. The treatment period was for 12 weeks. Note the specificity of Curaderm for the cancer cells and the regrowth of normal cells during Curaderm therapy. The clinical diagnosis was confirmed histologically by punch biopsy (f). After completion of the therapy histopathology determined that no residual cancer was present (g). Clinical assessment 5 years post treatment revealed that there was no recurrence.

extraction procedure to obtain the alkaloids in their native, natural state. I discovered that the alkaloids were not present as free alkaloids, but they were attached to certain sugars rendering them as glycoalkaloids. These purified glycoalkaloids were the substances in the eggplant that showed tremendous anticancer propertie[60, 61].

Further studies showed that if they were not purified to a certain standard their efficacy as anticancer agents dropped drastically. More investigational work was required to determine why this was the case. I then discovered that certain free sugars also present in the eggplant were affecting the anticancer properties of the glycoalkaloids. When these sugars were eliminated by further extraction the anticancer properties of the glycoalkaloids were optimal.

The "free" sugars were inhibiting the anticancer effects of BEC.

This means if you were to eat eggplant containing BEC you will also be ingesting the "free" sugars which nullify the anticancer properties of BEC.

Nature surely has some incredible unveiled secrets.

Chapter 8

COUNTERFEIT PRODUCTS

Various unscrupulous companies have preyed on the results of the extensive work done with Curaderm BEC5, and are making false claims that their products are equivalent or better than Curaderm BEC5. Little or no studies have been done with their products and these companies are cleverly attempting to deceive the public by associating my published work in their advertising material. It appears that there are no limits for supplying fraudulent information for what I assume is to become rich. These "parasites" have done everything possible to plagiarise and deliberately mislead the public for their own personal gains.

As described earlier in this book, it is not a simple matter of having glycoalkaloids in a cream or gel and assume that this is a treatment for skin cancer. Cancer is a serious condition. A tremendous amount of careful work was done to obtain these purified glycoalkaloids without traces of their inhibitors (interfering substances) from the plant materials. If this preparation is not properly completed, the end product will be useless, as experienced by patients who have been cleverly enticed to use counterfeit products. I have received numerous telephone calls, facsimiles, and emails from patients, all over the world, who have used these counterfeit products without success. The following is an example of a typical email received.

> "Greetings, I have used Curaderm in the past with great success. Last year I tried to order the product from ... and was told it was now called .... I waited 4 months and finally received two tubes of ... (supposedly Curaderm) with an offer to buy a book claiming to have the answer for skin cancer. Well, it didn't have the consistency of Curaderm, it didn't smell like Curaderm and quite honestly it was worthless. I was very impressed with the real Curaderm and would like to purchase some. If you could direct me to a reliable source I would be very grateful. Thanks"

This approach to blatantly pirate and plagiarise intellectual property and to simply deceive the public does not assist the genuine development of a product like Curaderm BEC5. Companies producing ineffective counterfeit products are disrespectful to science and they are tragically depriving the public of treatments for serious diseases, in this case a treatment for cancer.

Conclusion

Dermatologists, plastic surgeons and radiotherapists jointly manage non melanoma skin cancers. Such management usually involves surgery. The risks of surgical intervention are well known. Moreover, excision of these skin cancers from the facial area often involves reconstructive surgery, which can be both time consuming and costly. Hence an alternative, safe and efficacious method of treatment of such skin cancers that do not require physician or hospital attendance must be encouraged.

The benefits of Curaderm BEC5 has been recognized by the dermatological community and information on Curaderm BEC5 has been presented by invitation at the following international forums:

- World Congress on Skin Cancer (Zurich, 2001)
- European Academy of Dermatology (Geneva, 2001)
- British Dermatological Association (Leeds, 2001)
- British Dermatological Association (Cardiff, 2002)
- World Congress of Dermatology (Paris, 2002)

It was concluded that Curaderm BEC5 was a safe and efficacious method of treatment for non melanoma skin cancers and the treatment protocol did not require physician or hospital attendance.

The dermatologists involved with Phases III and IV of the clinical studies have commented that in their view and experience (Curaderm) BEC5 as topical application is a safe and effective ideal therapy for outpatient treatment. Hence (Curaderm) BEC5 is a much needed alternative to surgery for basal cell carcinoma. This is the commonest cancer in Caucasians worldwide and the prevalence continues to increase with an increasing ageing population.

Curaderm BEC5 results in ulceration of the lesion site during treatment. However, it is observed that post treatment the wound is quickly replenished with normal tissue.

The pictures of Curaderm BEC5 treated cancers in this book convincingly show that the cosmetic end result is magnificent. In the majority of cases when patients were followed up for several years after treatment with Curaderm BEC5 they could not distinguish where the cancer was!

Curaderm BEC5 is the method of choice for treating non melanoma skin cancers. Nevertheless, surgery is a needed procedure in selected cases where it can not be excluded that SCC metastases are suspected.

I can now finally reflect on the occasion that arose sometime ago in the 1990s (the "Mutilated Man"). With some satisfaction, respect and humbleness I feel that I have fulfilled one of the last wishes of a genuine nice couple who unselfishly encouraged me to make available a better treatment for skin cancer for the general public.

This I have accomplished!

BIBLIOGRAPHY

1. American Cancer Society. www.cancer.org

2. Canadian Centre for Occupational Health and Safety. www.ccohs.ca

3. E Health MD. http:/www.ehealthmd.com

4. Skincancer Foundation. www.skincancer.org

5. Cham, B. E. and Wilson, L. (1987). HPLC of glycoalkaloids from Solanum sodomaeum L. Planta Med. 53, 59-61.

6. Bajaj, K. L., Kaur, G. and Chada, M. L. (1979). Glycoalkaloid content and other chemical constituents of the fruits of some egg plant (Solanum melongena, L.) varieties. J. Plant Foods, 3, 163-168.

7. Chen, Z. and Miller, A. (2001). Steroidal Alkaloids in solanaceous vegetable crops. Horticul. Rev. 25. 171- 186.

8. Cipollini, M. L. (2000). Secondary metabolites of vertebrate – dispersed fruits; evidence for adaptive functions. Rev. Chil. Hist. Nat. 73. 421-440.

9. Ghazi, M. and Matthees, D. P. (1989). Use of ion-pairing reversed-phase liquid chromathography in separation of solanidine and solasodine. J. Chem. Exol. 15. 2661-2666.

10. Jones, P.G. and Fenwick, G.R. (1981). The glycoalkaloid content of some edible Solanaceous fruits and potato products. J. Sci, Food Agric. 32. 419-421.

11. Lequart, V., Goethals, G., Banoub, J., Villa, P. and Martin, P. (2004). An Improved Synthesis of Chacotriose. Chem. Let. 33. 444.

12. Morillo, M., Lequart, V., Grand, E., Goethals, G., Usubillaga, A., Villa, P. and Martin, P. (2001). Synthesis of peracetylated chaco-triose. Carbohyd. Res. 334, 281-287.

13. Nada, C., Nikolic, A., Mihajlo, Z., Stankovic, A. G., Dejan, Z. and Markovic, C. D. (2005). Liquid-liquid systems for acid hydrolysis of glycoalkaloids from Solanum tuberosum L. tuber sprouts and solanidine extraction. Med. Sci. Monit. 11(7). BR200-205.

14. Schreiber, K. (1968). Steroidal alkaloids: The Solanum group. In the alkaloids Vol 10, (Mansk, K., Ed.). Academic Press.

15. Cham, B. E. (1988). Monograph on the compound BEC. Drugs of the Future. 13, 714-716.

16. Daunter, B. and Cham, B. E. (1990). Solasodine glycosides. In vitro preferential cytotoxicity for human cancer cells. Cancer Letters 55, 209-220.

17. Cham, B. E. (1989). Curaderm (antineoplastic). Launched in Australia. Drug News and Perspectives 2, 112.

18. Cham, B. E. (1991). Solasodine glycosides: A new modality for cancer. In Proc. 2nd Oceania Symposium. Pp.30-36. Editor Mark S. Walker. Bioconcepts Publishing.

19. Cham, B. E. (1994). Solasodine glycosides as anti-cancer agents: Pre-clinical and clinical studies. Asia Pacif. J. Pharmacol. 9, 113-118.

20. Cham, B. E. (1993). Efficacy and mode of action of solasodine glycosides (BEC) on cancer cells. In Proc. 4th Oceania Symposium 0041-51. Editor Mark S. Walker. Bioconcepts Publishing.

21. Chataing, B., Christancho, N. B. and Usubillaga, A. (1998). Topical treatment of herpes simplex, herpes zoster and genital herpes with a mixture of Solanaceous glycoalkaloids. MedULA. Universidad de Los Andes. 7. 30-34.

22. Choi, E. and Koo, S. (2005). Anti-nociceptive and anti-inflam matory effects of the ethanolic extract of potato (Solanum tuberosum). Food Agri. Immun. 16. 29-39.

23. Hall, C. A., Hobby, T. and Cipollini, M. (2006). Efficacy and Mechanisms of α- Solasonine-and α-Solamargine-Induced Cytolysis on Two Strains of Trypanosoma cruzi. J.Chem. Ecol. 32. 2405-2416.

24. Kuo, K. W., Hsu, S. H., Li, Y. P., Lin, W. L., Liu, L. F., Chang, L. C., Lin, C. C., Lin, C. N. and Sheu, H. M. (2000). Anti cancer activity evaluation of the Solanum glycoalkaloid solamargine. Triggering apoptosis in human hepatoma cells. Biochem. Pharmacol. 60, 1865-1873.

25. Putalun, W., Taura, F., Qing, W., Matsushita, H., Tanaka, H and Shoyama, Y. (2003). Anti-solasodine glycoside single-chain Fv antibody stimulates biosynthesis of solasodine glycoside in plants. Plant Cell Rep. 22. 344-349.

26. Verpoorte, R. (1998). Exploration of nature's chemodiversity: the role of secondary metabolites as leads in drug development. Drug Discov. Today 3, 232-238.

27. Vijayan, P., Vinod Kumar, S., Dhanaraj, S. A., Badami, S. and Suresh, B (2002). In Vitro Cytotoxicity and Anti-tumour Properties of the Total Alkaloid Fraction of Unripe Fruits of Solanum pseudocapsicum. Pharmaceut. Biol. 40. 456-460.

28. Cham, B. E., Gilliver, M. and Wilson, L. (1987). Antitumour effects of glycoalkaloids isolated from Solanum sodomaeum L. Planta Med. 53, 34-36.

29. Cham, B. E., Daunter, B. (1990). Solasodine glycosides. Selective cytoxicity for cancer cells and inhibition of cytotoxicity by rhamnose in mice with sarcoma 180. Cancer Letters, 55, 221-225.

30. Amalfi, C. (2006). The little mouse who wouldn't say die. Cosmos Mag. 471.

31. Badami, S., Manohara Reddy, S.A., Kumar, E.P., Vijayan, P. and Suresh, B. (2003). Antitumour activity of total alkaloid fraction of Solanum pseudocapsicum leaves. Phytother. Res. 17. 1001-1004.

32. Chataing, B., Concepcion, J. L., Lobaton, R. and Usubillaga, A. (1998). Inhibition of Trypanosoma cruzi growth in vitro by Solanum alkaloids; a comparison with ketoconazole. Planta Med. 64, 31-36.

33. Chami, L.A., Méndez, R., Chataing, B., O'Callaghan, J., Usubillaga, A. and LaCruz, L. (2003). Toxicological effects of α-solamargine in experimental animals. Phyto Res. 17, 254-258.

34. Chang, L. C., Tsai, T. R., Wang, J. J., Lin, C. N. and Kuo, K. W. (1998). The rhamnose moiety of solamargine plays a crucial role in triggering cell death by apoptosis. Biochem. Biophys. Res. Commun. 242, 21-25.

35. Esteves-Souza, A., Silva, T. M. and Alves, C. C. F. et al. (2002). Cytotoxic activities against Ehrlich carcinoma and human K562 leukaemia of alkaloids and flavonoid from two Solanum Species. J. Braz. Chem. Soc. 13. 838-842.

36. Hsu, S. H., Tsai, T. R., Lin, C. N., Yen, M. H. and Kuo, K. W. (1996). Solamargine purified from Solanum incanum Chinese herb triggers gene expression of human TNFR1 which may lead to cell apoptosis. Biochem. Biophys. Res. Commun. 229, 1-5.

37. Evans, R., Cham, B. E. and Daunter, B. (1989). Letter to the Editor. Your Pharmacy, January, 1.

38. Cham, B. E. and Meares, M. M. (1987). Glycoalkaloids from Solanum sodomaeum L. are effective in the treatment of skin cancers in man. Cancer Letters 36, 111-118.

39. Cham, B. E., Daunter, B and Evans, R. (1992). Topical treatment of malignant and premalignant skin cancers by very low concentration of a standard mixture of solasodine glycosides. Clinical Digest Series. Dermatology. 1992.

40. Cham, B. E., Daunter, B and Evans, R. (1991). Topical treatment of malignant and premalignant skin cancers by very low concentrations of a standard mixture of solasodine glycosides. Cancer Letters 59, 183-192.

41. Cham, B. E., Daunter, B and Evans, R. (1990). Curaderm. Med. J. Australia. 152, 329-330.

42. Cham, B. E., Daunter, B. (1990). Topical treatment of pre-malignant and malignant skin cancers with Curaderm. Drugs of Today 26, 55-58.

43. Cham, B. E. (1989). Plants yield skin cancer cure. Austral. Technol. Rev. 2, 53.

44. Millward, M., Powell, A., Daly, P., Tyson, S., Ferguson, R. and Carter, S. (2006). Results of phase I clinical trials of Coramsine in patients with advanced solid tumours. J. Clin. Oncol. 24, 2070.

45. Nakamura, T., Komori, C., Lee, Y., Hashinoto, F., Yahara, S., Nohara, T., and Ejina, A. (1996). Cytotoxic activities of Solanum steroidal glycosides. Biol. Biopharm. Bull. 19, 564-566.

46. Roddick, J. G., Rÿrenber, A. L. and Weissenber, M. (1990). Membrane-disrupting properties of the steroidal glycoalkaloids Solasonine and Solamargine. Phyto. Chem. 29. 1513-1518.

47. Roddick, J. G., Weissenberg, M. and Leonard, A. L. (2001). Membrane disruption and enzyme inhibition by naturally – occurring and modified chaco-triose – containing Solanum steroidal glycoalkaloids. Phyto. Chem. 56, 603-610.

48. Jellinek, N. and Maloney, M. (2005). Escharotic and other botanical agents for the treatment of skin cancer: A review. J. Amer. Aca. Dermatol. 53. 486-495.

49. Moss, R. W. (1998). Herbs against cancer History and controversy. Equinax press, Inc. Brooklyn, N.Y.

50. Punjabi, S., Cook, I., Kersey, P., Marks, R., Finlay, A., Sharpe, G. et al. (2000). A double blind, multi-centre parallel group study of BEC-5 cream in basal cell carcinoma. Eur. Acad. Dermatol. Venereol. 14 (Suppl). 47-60.

51. Walsh, N. (2000). Promising Topical Therapy for Actinic Keratoses – Brief Article Dr S Punjabi. Uni. Liverpool. Family Pratice News. December 1 article.

52. Williams, D. G. (1995). The skin cancer cure nobody wants you to know about. Alternatives, 6, 17-22. Mountain Home Publishing.

53. Williams, D. G. (1995). The skin cancer cure so effective, it's being kept secret. Ingram, TX: Mountain Home Publishing.

54. Dr Calméz Ltd. www.curaderm.net

55. Sussman, L.A.E. and Liggins, D.F. (1996). Incompletely excised basal cell carcinoma: a management dilemma? Aust. NZ. J. Surg. 66, 276-278.

56. Cham, B.E. (2007). Solasodine rhamnosyl glycosides in a cream formulation is effective for treating large and trouble some skin cancers. Res. J. Biol. Sci. 2(7) 749-761.

57. Caramelli, B., dos Santos Filho, R. D., Sposito Ade, C. and Martinez, T. L. (1998). Effect of eggplant on plasma lipid levels, lipidic peroxidation and the reversion of endothelial dysfunction in experimental hypercholesterolemia. Arq. Bras. Cardiol. 71(1). 89.

58. Guimaraes, P. R., Galvao, A.M., Batista, C. M., Azevedo, G. S., Oliveira, R. D., Lamounier, R. P., Freire, N., Barros, A. M., Sakurai, E., Oliveira, J. P., Vieira, E. C. and Alvarez-Leite, J. I. (2000). Eggplant (Solanum melongena) infusion has a modest and transitory effect on hypercholesterolemic subjects. Braz. J. Med. Biol. Res. 33(9). 1027-1036.

59. Marchiori Praça, J., Thomaz, A. and Caramelli, B. (2004). Eggplant (Solanum melongena) extract does not alter serum lipid levels. Arq. Bras. Cardiol. 82.(3). 269-272.

60. Ono, M., Nishimura, K., Suzuki, K., Fukushima, T., Igoshi, K., Yoshimitsu, H., Ikeda, T. and Nohara, T. (2006). Steroidal glycosides from the underground parts of Solanum sodomaeum. Chem. Pharm. Bull. 54, 230-233.

61. Cham, B.E. (2007). Solasodine rhamnosyl glycosides specifically bind cancer cell receptors and induce apoptosis and necrosis. Treatment for skin cancer and hope for internal cancers. Res. J. Biol. Sci. 2(4) 503-514.

GLOSSARY

Actinic keratosis: a precancerous skin growth that occurs on sun-damaged skin often looks like a red scaly patch and feels like "sandpaper".

Anti-angiogenics: stops blood vessels from developing, thus reduces blood flow to the cancer.

Apoptosis: fragmentation of a cell into membrane – bound particles.

Basal cell carcinoma: the most common form of skin cancer that involves cells in the lower part, or base, of the epidermis, the outer layer of skin.

BEC: a constant, specific mixture of glycoalkaloids extracted from plant materials that possesses good anticancer properties.

Benign: non-cancerous, a growth that does not spread to other parts of the body or damage normal tissue.

Biopsy: removal and examination of cells or tissue under a microscope to check for cancer.

Carcinoma: cancer that starts in tissues that cover or line organs in the body.

Cell lysis: destruction of a cell.

Chemotherapy: treatment with anti-cancer drugs.

Clinical trial: a research study done on human volunteers to decide if a new treatment is safe and effective.

Curaderm BEC5: a cream formulation that contains BEC and is used for non melanoma skin cancers.

Curettage: a surgical method of removing diseased tissue with a curette, a sharp-edged instrument.

Curette: a spoon-shaped surgical instrument with a sharp edge.

Dermatologist: a medical doctor who specializes in treatment of skin cancer and other skin diseases.

Dermatopathologist: a medical doctor, generally a dermatologist with subspecialty training in skin pathology.

Dermis: the layer of skin, located under the epidermis.

Electrodessication: a surgical method of drying-out tissue by touching it with a needle-like electrode that passes electric current into the tissue.

Epidermis: the outermost layer of skin, which is in contact with the environment, located above the dermis.

Erythema: reddening of the skin.

Ex Vivo: outside the living body.

Glycoalkaloid: a sugar combined with a nitrogen containing substance found in plants.

GCMS: Gas Liquid Mass Spectrometer, a device that can measure very small quantities of a substance.

Haematological: blood related substances.

Histological: analyses of minute structure, composition and function of tissues.

Independent investigators: investigators who have done studies separately and are uninfluenced by other investigators.

In Vivo: within the living body.

Keratolytic agents: substances that soften and dissolve or peel the horny layer of the outer layer of the skin.

Laser: an electronic device that focuses light into an intense beam used in skin cancer surgery to cut or destroy tissue.

Localized: cancer that is limited to one small area of the body and has not spread.

Lymph nodes: clusters of tissue found in the underarms, groin, neck, and other parts of the body that help fight disease. When cancer spreads, they often trap cancer cells.

Malignant: a cancerous growth that may destroy nearby normal tissue and spread to other parts of the body.

Matrix metalloproteinase inhibitors: substances that prevent tumour spread and prevent blood vessels from forming.

Melanocytes: skin cells that produce a pigment called melanin and can change into malignant melanoma.

Melanoma: cancer that occurs in melanocytes and is the most serious kind of skin cancer.

Metastasize: the spread of cancer cells from the original tumour to distant parts of the body.

Mohs micrographic surgery: a method of treating skin cancer in which the cancer and as little normal tissue as possible is removed.

Mole: a small usually dark skin growth that develops from pigment-producing cells called melanocytes.

Monoglycosides: substances that have one sugar attached to them.

Pathologist: a doctor who helps diagnose disease by examining cells and tissues under a microscope.

Pharmacodynamics: the study of the action and effects of drugs.

Pharmacokinetics: the action of drugs in the body over a period of time.

Photodynamic therapy: treatment with drugs that kill cancer cells when exposed to a special light.

Precancerous: a growth that may eventually turn malignant and become cancerous.

Protocol: an explicit, detailed plan of an experiment.

Published information: unbiased, independent reviewed information such as scientific research that is printed in medical journals and is in public domain.

Radiation therapy: treatment that uses x-rays and other sources of radiation to kill cancer cells.

Recur: cancer that returns after treatment to the same site or a new site in the body.

Solasonine & Solamargine: glycoalkaloids found in Solanaceous plants such as the eggplant. The glycoalkaloids possess good anticancer properties.

Squamous cell carcinoma: cancer that occurs in squamous cells, which are specialized cells near the skin surface that produce protective keratin.

Topical chemotherapy: treatment with anticancer drugs in a cream or solution applied to the skin over a period of time.

Triglycosides: substances that have three sugars attached to them.

Tumour: any abnormal growth of tissue that can be either benign (non-cancerous) or malignant (cancerous).

Ultraviolet radiation: invisible rays in sunlight that cause suntan, sunburn, premature skin ageing, and most cases of skin cancer.

INDEX

T

U

V

W

X

About the Author

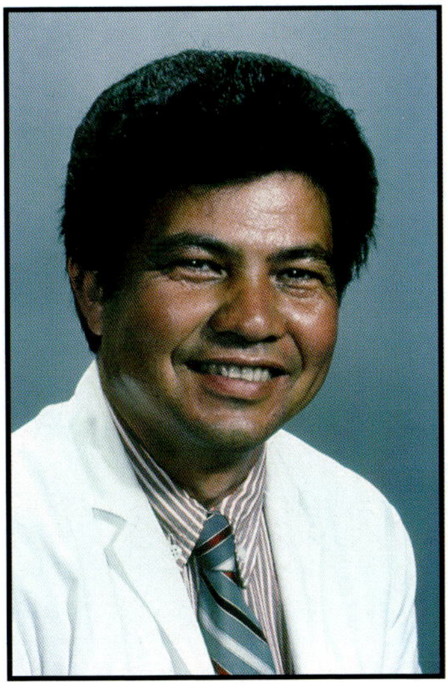

A member of many Scientific Societies, Dr. Bill Cham is frequently invited to speak at conferences on his research topics. His research interests cover a wide range of disciplines resulting in publications of over a hundred articles on topics ranging from pharmacology, iron metabolism, mineral research, lipidology and oncology. His research in lipidology starting from test tube observations, have led to clinical trials in the USA for the treatment of atherosclerosis, HIV, and AIDS.

His work in oncology has produced Curaderm BEC5 for the treatment of skin cancers. Human clinical trials in Australia are currently underway to establish whether BEC can also treat terminal internal cancers effectively.

Dr. Cham's research is acknowledged worldwide and many scientists are focused on extending his original discovery and research observations.

SmartPublications™

www.smart-publications.com

Please copy this page and mail or fax it to us at:

Smart Publications
PO Box 4667
Petaluma, CA 94955

Fax: 888-998-6889
Or call us, toll free, at 800-976-2783

We'll send you a free listing of alternative health and anti-aging product vendors. This comprehensive listing details where you can buy life-extending pharmaceuticals and anti-aging medicines without a prescription.

Name: ____________________
Company: ____________________
Address: ____________________
City/State/Zip: ____________________
Email: ____________________

What magazines do you subscribe to?

____

____

Age (optional): ____________________
Annual Income (optional): ____________________

Areas of nutritional medicine of particular interest:

____

____